THE KANDO TECHNIQUE

THE
KANDO
TECHNIQUE

JULIETTE &
MADELEINE KANDO

Thorsons
An Imprint of HarperCollins*Publishers*

Note

The moves and instructions presented in this book are not intended to be a substitute for medical advice. It is recommended that you consult your doctor before beginning this or any other exercise programme. The authors and publishers disclaim any responsibility for and injury, liability or loss in connection with the moves and advice herein.

Thorsons
An Imprint of HarperCollins*Publishers*
77–85 Fulham Palace Road,
Hammersmith, London W6 8JB
1160 Battery Street,
San Francisco, California 94111–1213

Published by Thorsons 1993
1   3   5   7   9   10   8   6   4   2

Juliette and Madeleine Kando assert
the moral right to be identified as
the authors of this work

A catalogue record for this book
is available from the British Library

ISBN 0 7225 2766 7

Typeset by Harper Phototypesetters Limited,
Northampton, England
Printed in Great Britain by
ScottPrint Limited, Musselburgh

Contents

Kando credits   6
Introduction: What is Kando?   7

1 FITNESS WITHOUT EXERCISE   16
2 SIMPLIFYING YOUR LIFE   21
3 WEIGHT LOSS   47
4 THE KANDO MOVES   54

   Hips, bums, tums and thighs   54
   Back, neck, shoulders and face   64
   Realignment   71
   Stance and balance   74
   Articulation – lying down   81
   Articulation – standing   97
   Strength and endurance   102
   Co-ordination and efficiency   110
   Recovery   113
   For partners   119
   For groups   126

5 KANDO IN YOUR LIFE   130

Appendix: Daily, weekly and monthly progress charts   134
Bibliography   139
Index   142

Kando credits

We would like to thank all the people who have so patiently and enthusiastically given their time both in a professional capacity as well as posing for many of the photographs.

Claudette Phillips	*Model/dancer/actress*
Jane Graham-Maw	*Senior editor*
Peter Chadwick	*Photographer*
Lucy Allen	*Designer*
Ros Saunders	*Design manager*
Barbara Vesey	*Copy editor*
John Dinsdale	*Book cover design*
Ellie Coyle	*Initial copy editor*
Iain Adam	*Adviser*
Miko Adam-Kando	*Equipment designer*
Tomi Adam-Kando	*One of our sons*
Kirsty Adam-Kando	*Cover model/gymnast*
Sandra & Adam Kinn	*Friendly neighbours and*
Martha & Jessica	*their children*
Mari Gaffney	*Illustrator*

Plus all our clients and friends who asked the right questions.

What is Kando?

Kando is total fitness without aimless, stressful, exhausting and time-consuming exercise. Kando is a technique for physical re-education which allows the body to use and express itself fully in day-to-day living. You are *not* lazy and fat, old, sluggish, ugly and clumsy. Your body has merely suffered lifelong negative habits from way back, when you first began to grow and move as a little baby. All your aches and pains, discomforts, complexes, doubts, fears, fatigue and lethargy may just be the result of a lifetime of incorrect movements and positions, of *negative physical habits*.

Now that the guilt chip has been taken off your shoulder you can regain a sound sense of self-esteem and begin to observe, to listen to, to converse with and to understand your body afresh.

Why not exercise?

While it is a sound natural instinct to improve oneself, to aim for physical and mental perfection in the well-known natural 'high' of transcendental, repetitious movement, a lack of up-to-date scientific evidence on the efficacy and safety of single training methods, the uncontrolled use of machines and the dumb copying of passing trends have failed many exercise enthusiasts. Some of the keenest fitness fanatics suffer from 'exercise addiction'. Caught in a double-bind, you don't get satisfaction from continuing yet suffer severe withdrawal symptoms and nagging guilt when you stop.

Ignorance and over-specialization in particular exercise methods are largely to blame for the bad name 'exercise' has acquired over the last decade. Experience has now shown (the hard way) that exercise often does people more harm than good. Unless you already enjoy perfect health and perfect posture (which do not exist and would eliminate the need for exercise), jogging and aerobics, for example, have proven to have an adverse effect, especially on the ankles and knees, and the lumbar and neck vertebrae, not to speak of the heart. Excessive weight training is known to lead people to aggressive, rude, in some cases even criminal behaviour. Single-handed racket sports such as squash, badminton, etc. can cause tennis elbows and other 'repetitive strain injuries' also found in football players and gymnasts who keep on performing with their best leg or side.

It seems then that people are either obsessed with doing exercise or guilt-ridden when they don't. Neither seems satisfactory. A better way to come to terms with your body is to accept it for what it is. The body you inhabit is the only one you've got. It is, as you will see, extremely well designed, friendly and accommodating, ready to serve you in the best possible way it knows how.

Back to the roots

Starting from the very roots of movement behaviour, four distinct forces can be identified which most affect our daily movements:

1. The constant downward pulling force of *gravity* which keeps us glued to the globe

2. *Genetically inherited* movements
3. *Specialized movements* acquired through learning
4. Unconsciously held *negative habits*

The first three are fine and can, with a little knowledge and practice, be used to our own advantage. Even gravity can be turned upside-down, as in yoga or by using a gravity invertor which literally hangs your body upside-down. Genetic evolution can be controlled. If you know, for example, that your grandmother had twisted toes, you will watch out what shoes to put on your daughter's feet to correct the condition. Specialized movements can be used to our advantage provided they are well shared and well balanced. There is no reason, for example, why actions such as cutting, brushing or even turning a screw should always necessarily be performed with the same hand. Ambidexterity plays an important role in the Kando technique. The force of *negative habits*, however, is becoming more and more worrying and is really what this book is all about: how to re-educate your movements and actions so that they enhance your skills rather than hinder them. But let us begin at the beginning, by looking at the effects gravity has on our daily movements.

Gravity

There is a delicate balance to be maintained between the pulling force of gravity and the body's ability to function efficiently. When your body is upright, as during most of its waking hours, the force of gravity is pushing straight down on the spine. Because the centre of gravity is high above the feet (in the pelvis), an upright human body is much more liable to be easily pushed over than is a four-legged creature such as a dog, for example. Balance, therefore, is one of our most vital endowments. Balance needs at all cost to be nurtured and reinforced. A standing posture has to be structured architecturally from the ground up and precariously balanced. When moving about, your body's balance has to readjust itself constantly, and with too much weight and poor posture this may all become very uncomfortable and tiring indeed. The Kando technique uses passive stretching, rolling, hanging and swinging moves to take advantage of gravity rather than suffer its constant downward-pulling force.

Genetically inherited movements – an original totality

At first, a baby makes fish-like movements by trying to propel itself with movements of the lower body only, or of the upper body only, just like a fish. Then, when the body and the nervous system mature, a baby exhibits 'snake-like' movements. These movements occur in the right arm and right leg, or left arm and left leg, in just the way a crocodile moves. Later yet, when the baby has reached a certain developmental level, the contra-lateral, 'primate-like' movement patterns emerge, whereby the right leg moves with the left arm, or the left leg with the right arm 'in opposition', as in crawling or walking.

In a young child, different body parts have not yet taken on their specialized functions in great detail. The left/right co-ordination of the legs for walking, the fine skills needed for manipulating objects, writing and pushing small buttons take years of practice to perfect. Now, obviously, humans need these skills to function in the very specialized way we do. But we pay a price for this specialization: we lose an original sense of totality.

The sense of totality, the charm found in pre-literate children as well as in the vanishing tribes of depleted rain forests, is almost totally lost in 'civilized' adults today. Much ritualistic dancing, for example, overwhelms those taking part: they are totally physically engaged, from the hair on their heads to their toes on the ground. A total absorption of the body in one activity is taking place. Children also show such total integration of the body. Observe children and notice how they have total confidence in their bodies. When children are trying to walk, write or draw, nothing goes spare, their body aura and presence are involved in the present action. Incidentally, when a child does not obey you, it is not out of disrespect or stubbornness. It is just because no faculty or 'body part' is able to give you attention at that moment. The child's whole being is fully occupied.

These basic genetically-acquired skills need not be lost in adults. Regaining some of them prevents so much discomfort, pain, ignorance, illness and premature ageing. At present adults experience totality through more extreme physical activities such as jumping on a large trampoline or parachute jumping, or in the more familiar act of sexual intercourse, or again through deeply-held religious beliefs or transcendental meditation. The reason these activities are exhilarating is because they put the brain into theta waves (higher consciousness) and give us a momentary feeling of completeness and total fulfilment. New, carefully targeted movements in comfortable environments can also give back the original sense of totality so badly needed for happiness and comfort.

Thus the original wholeness and balance in the human body is slowly being supplemented by more *specialized movements* which allow the young human to evolve into a 'co-ordinated, skilful adult'. Soon the child can walk upright without falling down all the time. Like an apprentice juggler, the child learns not to drop and break everything. Manual co-ordination becomes most finely tuned, later perhaps to be used in playing the piano, computer programming or micro-surgery. The child may or may not grow up to be an Olympic gymnast. Whatever the situation may be, in the beginning, children are taught basic manners of behaviour pertaining to their culture.

Before a child is ready for school, basic 'animal' and instinctive physical expression has been programmed out, to be replaced by the demands of a particular cultural environment. No longer is the child free to roam about like a happy little animal, he or she is now well on the way to becoming an adult – that is, a stiff, chairbound, upright and uptight creature who moves his or her hands, mouth and eyes quickly but uses very little of any other part of the body. This is illustrated by the anamorphic drawing of the human body in Figure 1. Its bodily parts are blown up or reduced to the degree to which they are used. An average person's use of daily movements entails mostly moving the hands, the face and head, walking a little, and sitting very much of the time.

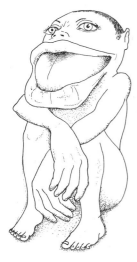

Figure 1:
Anamorphic body

Our bodies also react to this complex process of adaptation emotionally. We learn that it hurts when we fall down the stairs. We learn how to cover our heads and hunch our shoulders when we get hit by someone. Painful and unpleasant memories not only stick in our minds but in our bodies as well. People often cannot identify these 'emotional memories' verbally, yet they show in a permanently raised chin of defiance, the humble downward look of obedience, or the furtive look of suspicion. Movement therapy, which is not to be confused with physiotherapy, corrects embedded emotional features – such as, for example, an angry frown, a tense shoulder permanently raised in fear or the clenched fists of repressed aggression. As soon as the physical behaviour has been modified, the emotional trauma automatically disappears. Using both a mentally and a physically therapeutic approach to health and beauty problems attacks them from both extremes of human capabilities and guarantees the best results.

Our story

We were born in Budapest in 1943. Our family escaped communism in 1947, moving to Paris. At the age of seven we began ballet training, becoming professional dancers in our late teens. We each travelled the world in various dance companies for a decade or two and eventually settled down to start families of our own. Unfortunately, we quite accidentally landed on opposite sides of the Atlantic Ocean. Madeleine Kando (M.Ed.ADTR) became a dance/movement therapist in the mental rehabilitation unit of a Boston, Massachusetts, hospital. While I (Juliette) became a Fellow of the Institute of Choreology in London working as a dance/movement notator. The cocktail that became the Kando technique is a mixture of our respective professions blended with classical dance, yoga, T'ai Chi and a good deal of practical experience of caring for our bodies, learned in the daily practice of motherhood and teaching. The principles used here are not new or trendy. Most of them have been tried and tested over millennia.

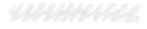

Classical dance

If classical dance can make a body supple, slender and expressive, we reasoned, then some of its principles could also be applied to daily functional movement. The training method of classical dance is based on rhythm, timing, balance, symmetry, line and aesthetic design. All these qualities conform with health and mechanical efficiency and can be put to good practice.

Yoga

The ancient discipline of yoga teaches that the body and the brain are one. Yoga uses movement and correct breathing to keep the body connected to the external world while it maintains top form. Unlike Western medicine, yoga understands that the process of life is not tangible, that it cannot be cut out of the body and put under a microscope. The essence of life, according to yoga, is made up of the ether and energy that flow through the body. Change, movement and forces circulate in and around the body, and these constitute life. By making the body more open and alert to these forces, yoga makes you feel more alive.

T'ai Chi

T'ai Chi is, again, a beautiful, ancient Eastern style of moving to engage the body in a slow, peaceful and gentle physical conversation with its environment and/or with one or more partners. Like many other forms of martial art, T'ai Chi teaches that maximum power comes from minimum effort. This we found an extremely welcome asset to a technique for tired bodies. Well-performed T'ai Chi movements flow continuously with tranquillity yet show great strength and stability in the body's centre and weight. It teaches that in order to be strong and balanced, the body needs to be firmly based, yet move as lightly as the wind.

Alexander

There are today an abundance of books published on the Alexander Principle and a whole network of qualified Alexander teachers throughout Britain and Europe all attempting to teach people to let go and allow the body to find its own 'natural' way of moving. Many of our clients are familiar with the Alexander Principle and have been practising obediently for many years yet their bodies are still mis-shaped and uncomfortable to them. A need has now arisen for a more up-to-date, immediately effective movement technique for 'every body'. Unlike the Alexander teachings, which originated in Alexander's own illness, the Kando technique originated in child development and approaches, skeletal alignment and gravity, inhibition, stress, direction etc. *not from a diseased point of view* in search for a cure, but from the most neutral and near-perfect body of a new-born child.

Motherhood

From the very beginning of motherhood, even during pregnancy, we wanted to keep our bodies in shape while raising our families. The only way it was possible to train and look after the kids at the same time was somehow to train with them at home. This turned out to become one of the most fascinating training periods of all times. What better teachers could we find than our own children, who had not yet been physically exposed to traumatic experiences? So our children helped us through a renewed phase of physical training: to move with the kids, like the kids. Fascinated by their natural determination, their courage and the ease with which they learned to move, we realized that they move naturally because they have none of the restrictions of ingrained movement patterns which are the result of a lifetime of physical and emotional tensions and discomfort.

Meanwhile, our contemporaries showed the usual worn-out-parents look and were tumbling towards middle-age with their bellies and moods hanging low. Morning sickness, ante- and postnatal depression, marital blues, hypertension, back aches, stiff necks, hunched shoulders and all the things that are supposed to come along with early parenting had always been completely alien to us. Our regular games with the children actually made our backs and arms stronger – as classical dancers our legs had always been the most powerful parts of our bodies until then. Our bodies now stretched us into new, long-forgotten positions which quite naturally made us once again supple, even more so than we had been in our dancing days.

Whenever the rare opportunity to see each other arose we shared our new movement experiences and communicated our ongoing research findings about adult physical behaviour. In the late 1970s we finally established two independent but very similar training programmes aimed at parents and children: *Toddlertone* in London and *The Children's Arts Corner* in Boston.

Kando and you

We are primarily concerned with creating space and a better way of moving in people's daily lives. The Kando technique demonstrates proper physical behaviour and shows in a fun and relaxed way how the body really can and wants to move. This requires an *ergonomically sound (body-wise) home environment* in which people can move well enough never to need to exercise.

The word 'exercise' does not feature in this book. Instead we deal with 'moves' which become an integral part of everyday life. Some may be practised while waiting for the kettle to boil, others can become integrated in your daily routines, and all moves are designed to be used in your actual, daily functioning. Comfort, space, light, ventilation, texture, clothing, colour and sound all play important roles in the technique, which is largely concerned with simplifying your life.

Major forces such as gravity, energy, genetics, acquired skilful movements and yes, even some negative habits can be changed around and used to your advantage. Feeling perfectly fit and alert without exercise becomes natural and a lot simpler than you'd ever have thought possible.

Fitness without exercise

It is not considered 'good form' to criticize someone's habits, so unless you are observant enough to notice poor habits in other people, you will never find them in yourself. Letting go of these perturbed-looking characteristics is like trying to give up smoking. They are addictive and so much a part of a person's identity that it would require an emotional amputation to get rid of them. Rather than trying to get rid of these negative patterns 'cold turkey', the Kando technique deals with them in an old Hungarian pedagogic (educationally effective) way: if you take something away you must offer something in return, then the loss is not missed. You learn to replace negative habits, be they physical or emotional, with *positive moves*. Before getting to specific moves, why not make yourself more comfortable right now by getting out of your chair and lying down on the sofa or the floor to read? Find a position in which you can more or less relax, and read on . . .

Passive stretching

Passive stretching is a very gentle way of gaining flexibility and improving articulation. This method is easy and pleasant and more effective than wildly pushing one's limbs about. For example, if you want to stretch the back of your leg right now, all you have to do is to straighten one or both of your legs and sit up straight against a wall. For any stretching to take place, three things must happen:

1. relaxation,
2. the use of an outside force such as gravity or weight, and
3. breathing.

Stretching demands *not doing* something rather than doing it. Muscles and tendons stretch all by themselves when they are allowed to relax. Passive, slow motion may be further encouraged by the position the body is in, to take advantage of its own weight slowly moving down with gravity. Force may be further increased by adding extra weight, in the form of loose ankle or wrist weights, or the weight of a partner's body or body parts in conjunction with manipulation or massage. So in the beginning, use only the natural force of gravity. Later on, when your body demands more thorough stretching, you may use additional weights carried passively by the body part concerned, or ask a partner to assist you by lending you some of his or her weight. (Don't get this confused with weight-lifting, which is *not* what this is about at all.)

Stretching is actually the wrong word for what is going on, as you are merely allowing your muscles and tendons to reach their natural length. It's really that simple: find the right position and let go, that's all!

No pain, just gain

When you feel a stretch pain you are feeling the reaction of the nerve-endings leading to muscles and tendons as those muscles and tendons get longer. The painful sensation is a tightness, a fearful resistance in your muscles to letting go, simply because the feeling is new and unfamiliar. Once your brain is able to tell your body parts that a stretch feeling is not a pain, then you can relax. Co-ordinated breathing releases the pain. Breathing also feeds the muscles with the additional oxygen they need in their new, extended position, and the sensation is very pleasant and gives great relief. Babies always laugh when you gently stretch their legs, for example. Spontaneous laughter is the best relief for tension. It is at this point of pleasure that you must stop. If you force the stretch further, it becomes unpleasant and will hurt tomorrow.

Caution: A fully stretched muscle carries some tension, like a stretched elastic. If you stretch too far, a piece of muscle can tear, snap, hurt like hell and take many months to heal. This is why stretching should always be done when the body is warm and relaxed, and take it very slowly, without bouncing or jerking. People often burp, pass wind, yawn, giggle or sometimes even cry after a good stretch, as it releases so many negative elements.

When should you stretch?

Chapter 4 describes many positions that you can use for passive stretching. You must stretch a little every day, when you wake up or *in* or after *the bath* or shower, when your body is warm. You can also stretch at any time during the day when you are stiff and tired, given the opportunity.

How often?

A stretch only has to be done once or twice until the extremity of a movement range has been reached. Too much stretching can cause problems: the muscles get hurt and retract further than when you started. A little stretching every day will get you a lot further than violently stretching once a week.

For how long?

You may remain relaxed in the positions for a few counts or a few minutes, depending on what your body has to say about it, but one thing should be borne in mind: when the body is placed in a new position, it will always make itself felt. People who never stretch perceive a stretch as a pain, a cracking joint as arthritis. A cracking joint is the sound of bones moving over each other when they have, for a time, not been moving much. It is nothing to worry about, as long as it doesn't hurt.

Use all your senses

The work at the Children's Arts Corner and Toddlertone led to some of the fundamental principles of this technique, namely:

1. *Combining the senses and faculties enhances learning*, and
2. *Basic needs are the same in all age groups.*

To put it more simply: the exhilaration you get from a good breath of fresh air feels the same whether you are 8 days or 88 years old. In both cases the body is designed to help the brain via the senses, and vice versa. All senses not only depend on each other but also, when used together, enhance the faculties. Each makes the others work better.

Put your sense of sight in perspective, for example, and discover how closely it is related to your daily actions.

Sight for balance

The sense of sight is most dominant, as it is used not only for looking, finding and identifying things but also in conjunction with balance. To test this out for yourself, try:

Balancing

1. Stand on one leg with your eyes open. This proves quite easy.
2. Now walk about to forget the sensation.
3. Try standing on one leg again, but this time with your eyes closed.

Good luck!

You have just learned about the sense of balance, and whether or not you have got one!

A learning technique works best when it is pleasant and enjoyable, when it gives satisfaction and a want for more. From a strong, centred alignment and a natural balance, moves develop that lead to a better shape, improved efficiency and more meaningful expression in the body. Like a child, the body then repeatedly asks: 'Do it again,' and learning becomes self-perpetuating. The result is that many physical complaints and emotional 'pains' can be self-cured, and ultimate fitness may indeed be attained without painful or strenuous exercise. We'll begin by simplifying your life to help you find comfort and freedom of movement.

Simplifying your life

In addition to inherited, habitual and emotional traces of your past experiences, your body is also confronted with current cultural and environmental dilemmas. Lack of space, bothersome clothing and ill-designed furniture, equipment and environments cause permanent, unnoticed discomfort which can lead to chronic injuries and syndromatic illnesses. An over-tolerance of perpetual discomfort has become part of life and is the root cause of many modern afflictions. As teachers, we have over the years dealt with many complaints, ranging from backache and migraine to rheumatism, depression and emotional trauma.

Your personal space

Each person's body occupies the space it needs from head to toe and as far as the limbs can reach. Although this amount of space is fixed by the size of your body and could be measured with a ruler, as soon as you begin to move and act, so your personal space also begins to change. The area around the body we use when moving, breathing, speaking, shouting or jumping may project itself into space beyond the physical body itself; it can change in size and density. You may act big or small and you can,

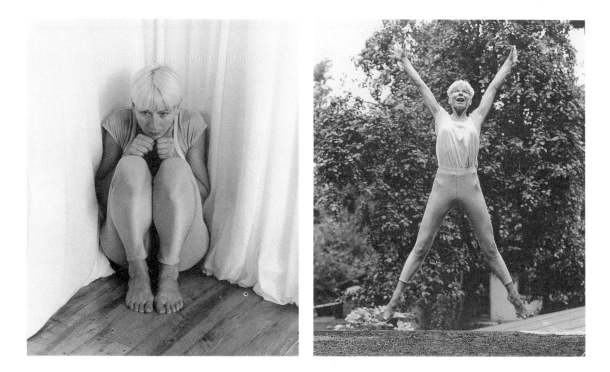

Figure 2:
Personal space –
two extremes

to a certain degree, control who or what enters or has an influence on your personal space. Expanding your personal space involves energy coming from the gut: the whole body, heart and soul. The allure of great actors and the grace of dancers depend on this. You too can do it and grow from within. To experience this for yourself, find out about the two extremes of your personal space.

Neither extreme is desirable for the body to be in for too long. It is necessary, however, occasionally to experience these two extremes in order to be 'physically informed' of one's potential.

Creating a 'body-friendly' home

It is important when designing a home to visualize the space with people and things in it and to imagine the traffic and movements the people will be making. Remember, a home has a finite volume (amount of space). For every item that *enters* the house, an equal amount of goods must *exit* or you begin to lose space. Walk around your living space moving your arms up and about and kicking the odd leg. How many walls, doors, tables and chairs are in your way?

Of all places, home is where the body must be allowed to move freely. Whether you live in a mansion or a bedsit, you can be king or queen of your own castle. Whether you are old or young, have a large family or live on your own, it doesn't matter. Moving freely at home includes daily stretching, relaxing, rebalancing and strengthening the body to face the crazy world outside. Health, beauty, balance and comfort go hand in hand. The first signs of illness are discomfort. When the body becomes used to being uncomfortable, it adapts and stops noticing discomfort. That is when you generally feel unhappy, listless, tired and moody. Passive discomfort is the root to many diseases today. The questions you should ask over and over again are:

- Am I really comfortable doing this or that action?
- Do I really need this or that gadget?

The answers will not come easily, because you may not be aware of real discomfort until you get a backache or other aches, become moody or angry for no apparent reason. The space in your home can either be filled, or it can be left empty. When it is filled, it stops being space. So the consumer who is quite tight for space has a choice: either to fill that space with things or to use the space for the body.

A clean floor

What you need

Many homes, especially small, newly converted flats, are just littered with doors and thin, hollow partitioning walls which, on reflection, you may not need or want. If you feel you'd rather have one large room than two small ones because the space that the wall and doors are occupying could be yours, then go ahead and knock the wall down. Of course, you must check that the wall is not weight-bearing, or the next floor would fall on your head and you might risk total demolition!

A free floor space at home must be large enough to allow your body to move in the horizontal position. It must be free of dirt and warm enough to lie down on. Minimum size: 6 sq ft (2 sq m) for one person.

A full-length mirror

The large mirror (preferably 5 ft/1½ m long) adds visual space to your environment. Place the mirror near a window – this will give you double the amount of natural light. A full-size mirror is as essential in the home as a cooker or bathtub. You need it to correct and check your posture, not only when you are working on your body but at all times. As you pass the mirror you can catch yourself stooping or hanging or even making an ugly expression. There is nothing wrong or vain about keeping one's physical habits in check. In addition to this large mirror, place a smaller mirror at an angle somewhere on an opposite shelf or surface. This permits you to view your whole body from the back and sides. This may seem rather voyeurish, but how else are you going to correct your posture, unless you begin looking at it from all sides?

Clear all clutter

The problem faced in many homes is a cluttering dance of objects. A choice must be made: is this space mine, or does it belong to an object? A simple rule can be applied: if the object in question has not been used or looked at in more than two years, has been forgotten altogether and has no sentimental, visual or functional use any more, then get rid of it. Any object that can be discarded, regardless of its original price, gives a little more space in the home: say 'Adieu, thank you for your services, good bye, enjoy your next owner.' Visual clutter is one of the worst irritants. Depending on how much space there is in the home, it is always a good idea to have as much clear visual space as possible. Imagine you are a film director or photographer and you are using your home as location for a movie or photography shoot. The subject in the picture is yourself plus all the other people that will frequent your space. The first thing a director or photographer does is to look at the background. Anything vaguely unrelated to the subject or to the visual composition of the picture must be removed. Build a few shelves for the things you want to see and a few fitted cupboards for the things you want to use but not look at all the time.

Furniture can seriously damage your health

Poorly designed appliances and heavy, immobile chairs, desks and beds can all seriously damage your health. Well-made furniture far outlasts a human lifespan, so one would think that if you had a chair that was really comfortable, you would never need another. Yet nothing seems further from the truth in our world. This 'need' for new furniture is in fact a manifestation of physical discomfort. When you go out to buy a new easy chair, your body is seeking a change of posture, not a change of chair. Another chair will only keep the body in a *similar* sitting posture and not satisfy its need for radical change. The consumer doesn't understand this and keeps on buying new chairs without ever really being comfortable. Getting off the furniture makes you get to know your body and teaches you how to feel good, at home in your own skin with very little else.

Dressing for comfort

As you begin to move more freely, your body will become more fussy about the items of clothing and accessories it is prepared to tolerate. In the end, your daily dress style will be so comfortable that it will no longer be necessary to change into 'special gear' for your moving sessions, as you will be moving freely full time. While we are not asking you to turn up in a track suit at the office tomorrow morning, when you are at home, relaxing or entertaining, you can begin taking off any articles of clothing and accessories that hinder freedom of movement. How many unnecessary items of clothing are you wearing right now?

No shoes if possible

More and more people are adopting the cleaner and healthier custom of wearing shoes outside the home only. If you can't get people to take their shoes off at the front door, at least have a few rooms that are shoe-free. Shoes protect the feet from cold and dirt outside, but in the house they only squash the feet, prevent them from airing and hinder freedom of movement in the toes, which is so vital for balance and circulation. Shoes are not shaped like feet. Take them off when you can.

Definitely no high heels

One of the reasons why high heels came into fashion is that they lift and tighten the calf muscle and accentuate the tilt in the pelvis, making the buttocks protrude.

High heels have a number of disadvantages: they force the weight of the body to slide forward into the shoe, which then presses on the toes causing corns, bunions, hammer toes, bruising and all sorts of nasty side-effects. The raised heel shortens the calf muscle, which is attached to the Achilles tendon (the hard tendon that connects the heel to the calf). Unless counter-stretches are applied, a permanently shortened muscle remains tight even when the shoes are taken off, and this then reduces the depth to which the knees can bend when standing. Stiff knees diminish the degree of bounce in the legs, which, in turn, hinders running and jumping actions and is over-compensated by a tipping of the pelvis and a deepening of the spinal curves.

If the base of a construction (in this case the sole of the foot) is leaning inefficiently, it is bound to affect all the parts supported by it. Shortened calf muscles reduce mobility in the knees, which pulls the pelvis forward, which in turn affects the torso, upper body, head and neck. This results in a posture in which the belly hangs forward and down while the backside is pushed out and up. If left uncorrected, the distortion continues into the upper part of the body, neck and head.

Many of our clients have admitted they can no longer walk on flat shoes, it actually hurts them. A pain is usually felt on the shin when a high-heel wearer tries to wear flat shoes for the first time. This pain is perfectly explainable and goes away in a few days. The muscles on the shin have to work a little harder to flex the

Figure 3: a) high-heeled posture with increased curvature; b) normal posture

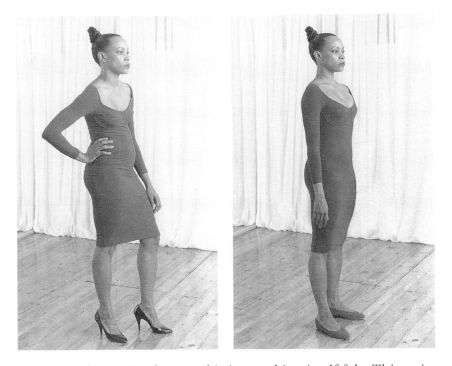

foot as each step is taken, and is just making itself felt. This pain can be relieved with massage and is only temporary. High-heel wearers often think they have a big belly and bottom when in fact all they are doing is holding their pelvis incorrectly. As soon as the position of the pelvis is rectified, so immediately the belly and bum also disappear. So don't wear high heels unless you are dressing up for a special occasion and really feel you must. Encourage your feet to be in a natural position and everything will soon turn back to normal: your calf muscles will lengthen again, your knees will straighten, your belly and bum will disappear and you will grow taller.

More no-nos of fashion for freedom of movement

- Underpants have tight elastic waist and groin bands. Wear boxer shorts or loose cotton leggings instead.
- Belts stop proper breathing.
- Bras prohibit breathing. Their shoulder straps cause indentations and tension in the shoulders of heavy-breasted women. They discourage muscle growth for holding the breasts in place in young women. Only wear them when you have to run or jump.

- Shirts and ties make people choke and inhibit movement in the neck and full circumferential vision. Hence perhaps the narrow, short-sighted views of those who wear them as a habit.
- Shoulder pads shorten the neck line and make you look frightened.
- Suits are shoulder-padded, heavy and warm. They hide the shape of the body and restrict freedom of movement.
- Scarves rub against the skin and aggravate neck wrinkles. Only wear them when you are cold.
- Watches and jewellery – the skin doesn't like hard, metal objects.
- Wearing shoulder bags is really asking for trouble. It is, by the laws of gravity, impossible to carry a shoulder bag without lifting the shoulder from which it is hanging. Try to hang a shoulder bag on a relaxed shoulder and it will fall off. A permanently raised shoulder not only gives you neck tension, which shortens your neck and can give you headaches, it also puts your whole posture off-balance and gives you a frightened look. Shoulder bags should be abandoned forthwith, unless worn across the chest, which is OK for men but less comfortable for well-endowed women.
- Handbags are containers of many unnecessary personal items. A few keys, credit cards and a little cash can fit safely into an inside pocket. Try, for once, walking along the streets without clutching a handbag and see how embarrassed your hands will be at first until your arms learn once again to swing freely and help you balance in walking and running.
- Glasses can weaken eyesight and prevent free movement of the head, while contact lenses irritate the eyes and can also weaken eyesight (for alternatives, read *The Natural Face Book* (Thorsons) or *Better Eyesight without Glasses* (Thorsons)).
- Hats make you bald as they prevent light and air getting to the roots of your hair.
- Gloves prohibit sensitivity in the fingers.
- Umbrellas are always left behind and lost.
- Long coats are often too heavy and restrict the length of your stride when walking.
- Tampons, coils, etc. can cause infections. This is especially true when women forget to take a tampon out, as has been known to happen.

Dress for moving

We have been in Paris, London, Amsterdam, Berlin, Tokyo, New York and Los Angeles. We have seen the fashion, the prices and the hype and come right back home to Arlington Heights or the market in Kilburn High Road for a very simple, cheap, comfortable wardrobe consisting mostly of adaptable 'leisure wear' applicable to men, women and children alike:

Basic wardrobe

- leggings
- shorts
- cotton vests
- cotton T-shirts
- plain knitted cotton sweaters
- some silks for posh occasions
- a few short jackets (with inside pockets so you needn't carry a handbag)
- sandals
- sneakers
- 'snuggle socks' (thick socks for home wear)
- dressing-up gear for special occasions (this may include many no-nos – as long as it all comes off after the event)

Movement and style

More than your style of dress, the way you move reveals your sexuality, character and mood. Masculinity or femininity is carried in the body's movements, not in clothes. It is *not* clothes that maketh a man (or woman). Stylishness is not *what* you wear, it's *how* you wear your clothes. The most expensive designer wear, hair-do and jewellery can look hideous if you don't carry yourself well or if you are frowning. When you are comfortable, at ease, you are ready to show your style. Style is a mark of health and personality and fits the body's own virtues: simplicity, humility, efficiency and adaptability. Be yourself and be happy with yourself. If you feel good and comfortable, being attractive will follow automatically.

Body-friendly equipment

The following simple pieces of equipment and teaching aids can be home-made ever so simply.

A floor mat and soft bolsters

If your floor is too hard, you need a mat. Soft bolsters are very handy to 'fill up' stiff curves in the body, for example under the knees, in the lower back or behind the neck, when you are sitting or lying down.

A soft, light, easily washable mat and bolsters can be made simply and cheaply. The mats may be used individually or piled up to meet different needs. All you need is:

Nine pillow cases in your favourite colours.
1. Measure the pillow cases.
2. Buy twelve 2 in-/5 cm-thick pieces of foam cut to the size of the pillow cases.
3. Put the pillow cases around nine pieces of the foam. These are your mats.
4. Roll up the three remaining pieces of foam.
5. Stick packaging tape around each roll to keep the edges of the foam together. These are your bolsters.
6. If you can sew, make a proper cotton cover for your bolsters. If you can't, improvise by sliding each bolster into the cut-off leg of an old pair of cotton leggings or into a long sock, tying the end together.

Hard bolster

Sometimes the spine likes to roll about or be on a slightly harder bolster. Slide a piece of wooden dowelling inside one of the soft bolsters before putting the cover on. A hard bolster is very effective for getting stiff vertebrae back into place, or as a prop behind the lower back when sitting in a chair.

To make it you will need:

- A piece of dowelling 1 in/2½ cm in diameter, cut to the width of your foam.

Rolling board

The rolling board is for ironing out the spine. It gives you a lovely releasing and tickling massage which will make you giggle despite yourself.

You will need:

- 24 pieces of dowelling approximately 1 in/2½ cm in diameter (this is quite a bit thicker than a broom stick), each piece cut to the *width* of one of your soft mats, plus
- 2 pieces of corner edging ¾ in/2 cm wide (this must be less wide than the dowelling), each cut slightly longer than the *total length* of all 24 pieces of dowelling laid side by side.
- 2 pieces of corner edging slightly longer than the *width* of your mats.

1. Screw the corners of the edging together to make a loose frame.
2. Lay the pieces of dowelling side by side on a smooth floor.
3. Put the frame on top of the dowelling. Your rolling board is finished.

Figure 4:
a) dowelling;
b) corner edging;
c) rolling board

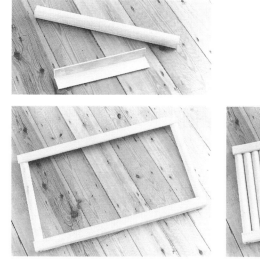
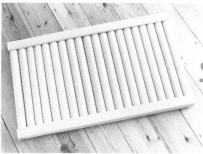

Ankle and wrist weights

Small weights, up to 2½ kg each, are often used in loose, throwing movements to loosen the joints and increase power in the legs or arms. You may purchase them at any good sports shop.

Canvas straps

Straps help you reach those parts you can no longer reach. They may be obtained at sports shops or boating and camping shops. Or, if you can sew, you can easily make strong straps from old cotton clothes that were due to be jumbled.

Small beauty pillow

Roll up a face towel from both ends inward. Use this to give you support at the sides of your skull and at the nape of your neck.

Figure 5: Small beauty pillow

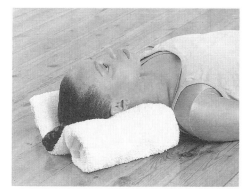

Five-toed 'snuggle socks'

The five-toed 'snuggle sock' works wonders for people who suffer from corns, bunions, hammer toes, or any problem with their feet. These socks keep the area between the toes dry, which prevents sweating and athlete's foot, and also encourages your toes to spread. You can make them by sewing four seams into a pair of very large and wide cotton socks to create a separate space for each toe. Wear them at home to improve all foot conditions and also to widen your stance and thereby improve your stability and balance.

Extra-wide trapeze

Hanging and swinging by the arms like a monkey lets down tension in the spine and legs and is very rejuvenating. If you build a trapeze into your living space, you are more likely to use the opportunity to hang once in a while. So why not create that facility, ready to fulfil your desire to hang, swing, perhaps even fly a little? The trapezes sold in shops are always too narrow to allow correct use of the arms, so we suggest you simply make your own. It will also cost you less.

You will need:

- A piece of dowelling measuring 4 ft/1.2 m long by 2 in/5 cm in diameter.
- 2 strong hooks
- 2 strong ropes, about 5 ft/1.5 m long each, depending on the height of your ceiling, and adjustable in length with the attachments necessary to
    a) attach ropes to hooks, and
    b) attach ropes to trapeze.

The hooks should either be bolted into the beam of your ceiling (if it is a metal beam) or screwed in (if it is a wooden beam). The hooks should be 3 ft/90 cm apart, to meet the dowelling 9 in/20 cm in at either end.

Caution: Make sure you get rope of the correct thickness and the proper bits and pieces. Make sure the dowelling is no thinner than 2 in/5 cm in diameter. Try to ask the shop assistant at the timber or boating shop when you buy the equipment. You are doing all this at your own risk.

Hammock

The hammock should be hung up in a tree in your garden. There is nothing more soothing than gently swinging and relaxing outdoors, listening to the sounds of nature and feeling a clean breeze of air across your closed eyes. If you haven't a garden but you have a balcony, put it there. If you've neither, put the hammock indoors, near an openable window.

Giant bolster

The giant bolster is wonderful for rolling over, leaning back on or straddling. Put it under your knees at night and it will prevent you from rolling over onto your side while you are asleep. A beauty sleep on your back saves the face many crinkles and wrinkles.

You will need:

- A 4 ft/1.2 m long piece of plastic drain pipe, the widest width you can get (which is about 9 in/20 cm in diameter).
- A piece of foam 5 in/15 cm thick, 4 ft/1.2 m long and 1½ ft/45 cm wide.
- Cow gum or any rubber-solution based glue.

1. Cover the two long edges of the foam with ample glue and let it dry for seven minutes or longer, until it feels tacky.
2. Wrap the foam around the pipe so that its long edges meet and stick together.
3. Tape the ends while allowing to dry.
4. Make a tight-fitting cotton cover.

Angled mirror

The image you see daily in the mirror is not the same as the image other people see. Over-familiarity with your own image prevents you from seeing what you really look like. To help you see your profile and your 'inverted' face as seen by outsiders, fit an angled mirror somewhere in your house.

You will need:

- Two pieces of mirror, ⅓ in/3 mm thick and 9 x 9 in/20 x 20 cm large. Ask in your local glass or DIY shop and they will cut these two pieces, polish the edges and give you a special glue to stick them onto the wall.

Find a free corner somewhere in your home. There, at head height, stick the two bits of mirror on the wall at right angles to one another.

You might even become inventive and design additional 'thingies' that will help your body become more comfortable. We welcome any 'tried and tested' solutions to your problems so that we may include them in future editions of this book. So *do* write to us with any problems you've come across or any new inventions and contributions.

Mothering hands for comfort

Throughout the moves given in the technique, don't be afraid to use your hands on the parts of your body that feel sensitive. Regard your hands as the 'mothers' of your body. They are strong, caring and most sensitive. Laying the warm, hollow part of your palm on a sore knee, for example, or on the solar plexus (the midriff) when you're feeling distressed, is most healing. The strong energy carried in the hands travels into more needy parts of your body. Your hands can also 'listen out' for little feelings and help you get better through self-massage.

Self-massage

Like a cuddly brown bear who scratches its back against a tree, self-massage can be most satisfying provided two things are borne in mind:

1. The purpose of massage is to relax and allow body parts to *be moved* passively.
2. When muscles act (are at work) they are contracted and cannot relax. The wrong type of self-massage would make you more tired than before you started.

If, for example, you decided to rub the painful right side of your neck with your right hand, then you are not going to get very much relief. Why not? Because while your right hand is busy rubbing the pain in the neck, your whole arm is contracting the

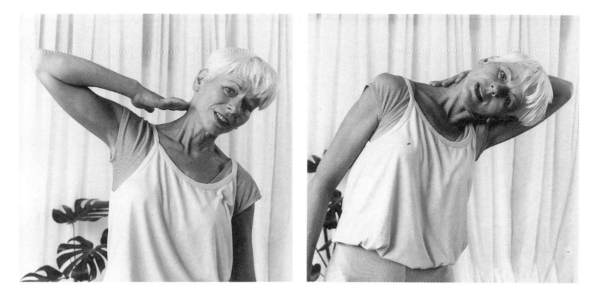

Figure 6:
DIY neck massage:
a) incorrect;
b) correct

very muscles (those above the shoulder) it is trying to relieve from tension. So think before you act. The position in which you hold your head is in this case crucial. If your head is held up, your neck is contracted and cannot relax, so no amount of rubbing will do anything at all. Your pain will only increase, as will your irritability.

In this way you can massage any part of your body provided the body part in question is fully relaxed and passive and you accompany the massage with soft movements and deep breathing.

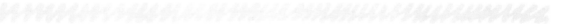

Ergonomics

Ergonomics deals with design to fit bodies. It originated as part of defence research and is used today mostly in industry to design the most 'body-friendly' tools, machines, work stations and environments. Ergonomics now plays an important role in engineering, psychology, the nuclear power industry and computer technology. It has also been cited in lawsuits made against manufactured products and work stations that are so badly designed that they've caused injuries or illnesses such as M.E. (myalgic encephalomyelitis, also known as post-viral fatigue syndrome) or R.S.I. (repetitive strain injury).

From the point of view of the private user/consumer, ergonomics still has a long way to go. Most people have never even heard of the word ergonomics, let alone begun to recognize its merits. Manufacturers of consumer and utilitarian goods seem to regard humans as either upright, sitting or lying-down creatures who don't move very much. Things are designed not to fit our bodies, but to fit a square box which can be easily stacked in a lorry. Then, industry designs more new gadgets to fix up our bodies damaged by previous gadgets in the form of exercising machines and all the leisure-market paraphernalia that comes along with that. Do we need it all? Our bodies certainly don't.

Early planning can help to create the ideal home, but only practice, movement and time will tell if you've done the right thing. While constantly adapting and seeking to improve behaviour, changes in our personal surroundings are inevitable. If something is bugging you, change it. Don't be afraid to change your mind. Don't fix things too permanently; that way they can easily be changed again. Allowing for the possibility of change gives you more freedom of movement. Certain fittings and appliances such as those in the kitchen and bathroom, as well as audio and video equipment, etc., are permanently plugged in and must therefore remain in place. These features, however, can all be fitted to save your body much repeated inconvenience, discomfort and irritation.

Don't be afraid of being 'peculiar'

Standard modes and appliances, mass-produced goods such as 'fitted kitchens', bedrooms, bathrooms, etc. are designed for an average consumer who looks like the model in the glossy catalogue. Don't consider yourself average. Each and every body is a very special individual, with its own personal measurements, movement patterns, habits and needs. Buy only the things that are 'user-friendly'. This will force the marketplace to become extremely competitive and inventive, and people will no longer feel like powerless targets of a consumer society. Forget standard recommended measurements – centimetres, millimetres, inches and tape measures. Use your body and its meticulously worked out proportions to establish the exact and correct measurements for all your home fittings and made-to-measure pieces of furniture. Do not think in terms of figures and numbers, statistics and averages. Look at your body and feel its reactions. This allows you to find comfort and economy in action.

Request and demand from shops, manufacturers, builders and your work place that they supply you with what you want, with what fits your very own body. Changing the height of a kitchen sink, computer keyboard or monitor is not a lot of hassle when you come to realize that it is as important as buying the right size shoes.

Ergonomic hints in the living-room

The amount of strain used in holding up one's head when watching a movie is equal to holding five bags of sugar on an outstretched arm for the same length of time. If a physical practitioner asked a patient to hold a position for such a length of time, he or she would be sued for malpractice. Yet people do it to themselves all the time. When you think you are relaxing, in the cinema, at the theatre, in a concert hall or pub, your neck and shoulder muscles are working all the time. Nesting daily by the television in the same position distorts your body slowly but gradually.

Figure 7: Couches built into your body

• Try to change sides and positions as frequently as possible, and

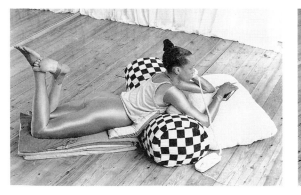
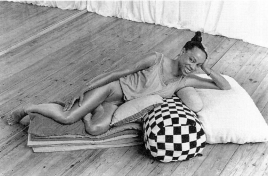

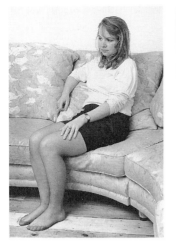

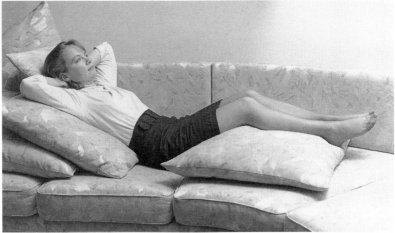

Figure 8: TV-watching positions:
a) incorrect;
b) correctly supported

learn to lounge horizontally with a few mats, cushions and bolsters which can help you support your body *and head* in many different, comfortable lounging positions.

- Place the television set high up above your bed to allow a healthy corrective position. For example, if you find that the best part of the day is spent sitting, or curling forward, a large cushion under your spine and a few more under your knees will soon straighten you up. If you accidentally fall asleep, your body will find its own corrective movements. Special nets can be obtained from the Kando catalogue (see back of the book).

Ergonomic hints in the kitchen

- Use low-placed cupboards for things you use less often, such as vases, rarely used kitchen gadgets, etc.
- Place heavy duty pans, etc. on high surfaces – perhaps the top of the refrigerator – to save you lifting heavy things from the floor.
- Put all the things you use daily, such as plates, cups etc., on surfaces that can be reached without having to bend down.

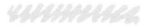

Work surfaces

All kitchen tops and sinks, bathroom sinks and other surfaces, gadgets and knobs should be built at a height that doesn't force your body to bend down unnecessarily to reach them. The rule of thumb for measuring a worktop is to measure from the floor up to your hip bone (the top part of the pelvic bone, where your waist begins). This is also near the place where your elbow bends naturally, and is the correct height for a work surface when the body is standing upright.

Surface too low

Anything lower than hip-bone height forces your spine to bend forward for each action, be it cutting bread, picking up a plate or anything else. This will unnecessarily strain your back. Bending down requires your body to lower itself and will either strain your back or legs or both. Bending the legs is much better for posture, but a lot of people cannot do this if their knees are too stiff and their thigh muscles too weak. There is a right and wrong way to bend down, but even when you bend down correctly it requires a lot of effort from your leg muscles. If sinks and worktops are too low and cannot be changed immediately, it is always better to take a wider stance (which lowers the body height and increases balance) *and*, if necessary, also bend the knees a little (second position demi plié) rather than keeping the feet together and excruciatingly bending over the spine.

Surface too high

A sink or work surface that is too high is equally uncomfortable. If, for example, the taps in the sink are higher than elbow-height, all the water will run up your sleeves every time you wet your hands. If you are cutting vegetables or screwing something down on a surface which is too high then you cannot put enough downward pressure, so the action is weak and demands an overload of muscle power in your arms and shoulders, creating unnecessary tension. These may all seem minor disadvantages, but when a movement is constantly wrong, over a long period of time, it becomes irritating, feels clumsy and produces aches and pains everywhere. Yet the situation can be so easily remedied.

Take the trouble to stand on one or more telephone books or a small box so that your hip bone and your elbows are at the right height and your manipulative skills will improve in a flash. Children are always happy with this solution. Short people can use the hint to save them feeling clumsy and weak. The additional benefit is that many mundane, unpleasant tasks will suddenly become a piece of cake to do.

At the office

Usually, when the body is unwilling to do an action, there is something wrong. But the wrong is not necessarily in the action, the wrong may be in the body. When doing desk work, the body is trapped in a static position which is becoming increasingly uncomfortable as the hours go by. It may walk about to the canteen at lunch time, go to the loo a couple of times and lean over someone else's desk, but on the whole the movement vocabulary used in offices is restricted to the following:

- sitting
- standing
- walking
- leaning
- manipulation (typing, writing).

These moves are affected by:

- eye strain
- ear strain
- air deprivation
- natural light deprivation
- noise strain

After lunch, the stomach is full. It would like to lie down and rest to digest its food, but this can't be done. The body is back at its desk, folded at the waist and pelvis, squashing its contents, which would like to flow freely through the digestive system. It's really better not to have lunch but to go for a walk or lie down instead.

Desk work

What exactly happens when you are sitting, working at a desk? Working at a desk limits the body to a very small number of positions, none of which are really comfortable for very long.

The upper part of the body leans over the desk supported by arms, elbows or hands. If you are engaged in a telephone conversation or taking down notes by hand, you are usually leaning to one side, and your head tilts accordingly depending on whether you are right- or left-handed. A permanent 'desk-writing' posture is adopted and becomes established.

While maintaining an imbalanced posture over many hours, weeks, months and years of working at the same job, the body is not aware of any immediate tension or discomfort until this manifests itself when headaches, a stiff neck and shoulders and back injuries emerge in protest. What has happened over the years is that muscle tension has taken over the job of the skeleton in maintaining the body upright. Bones become weaker and muscles turn hard, like marble pillars, pressing on nerves and further distorting the imbalanced skeletal structure. In addition, the eyes and ears will, later on in life, also develop an imbalance and become weaker as a direct result of constantly imbalanced sitting.

What is going on below the desk? In Figure 9 we see that the seat area supports the upper body on the chair and has to adjust its movements slightly but constantly, every time a movement is made upstairs (above the desk) by the arms, head, etc. The waist, hips and thighs are making compensating movements to keep the body in balance. To facilitate all these movements, the pelvis should be straight so that the trunk is supported by the sitting bones and not the tail.

So far so good, the pelvis is supported by the chair, but the lower legs are still weighing on the ankles and feet, which don't really get much relief at all. Legs shift, cross, uncross, kick a little. Feet twitch with discomfort. Crossing the legs takes the weight off one foot temporarily but only to give it to the other foot, so that's no help. Meanwhile the heart, whose job it is to circulate blood throughout the body, has to pump blood to the brain and down to the weighed-down toes stuck inside tightly laced, well-polished shoes. No wonder a person is tired after a day's work at the office.

The work station

1. The seat of a chair should be at knee-height (where your legs bend), so that your feet can rest flat on the floor.
2. Your spine must rest on the sitting bones (two protrusions under your bum), not the tail bone. Prop something behind your lower back if you have a tendency to sink into your spine.
3. When you are seated the desk top should be at waist-height, where your elbows bend, to allow your forearms and hands to rest horizontally (without having to lift your shoulders!) This is also the correct height for using a keyboard.
4. The height of a computer monitor (and this is usually where things go drastically wrong) should be at *eye level*, to allow your spine to be held fully erect and balanced.

Figure 9: Sitting on a chair:
a) incorrect;
b) correct

Take the trouble at work to rearrange your work station to fit your own body measurements. A good office chair allows for the

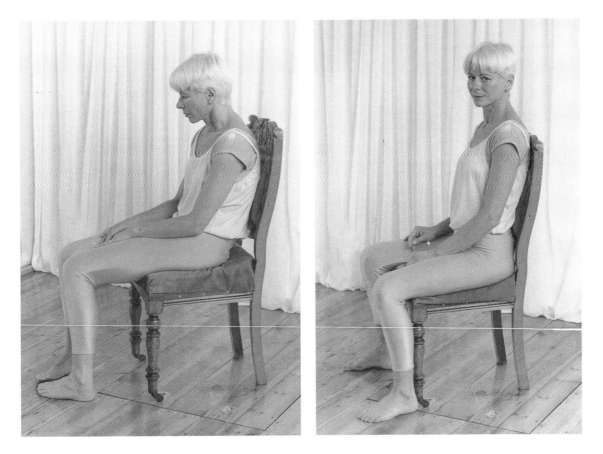

necessary height adjustments. It is often enough to put a cardboard box under the monitor to elevate its height to match your vision.

Choreography

In addition to placing sinks, worktops and appliances at physically convenient heights, it is, in the long run, a great advantage if you can think through the daily choreography of the movements you have to make in the home or work place to avoid unnecessary travels between sinks, cookers, cupboards, shelves, etc., and to restrict too much bending, turning and twisting. Increased traffic in a confined space is often the cause of many little accidents which can be easily avoided with just a slight modification of where things are placed.

For example, it makes sense to place the dishwasher near the sink and the cupboards in which the plates and things are to be put away. But the dishwasher need not be on the floor, as bending down to put each plate in is more strenuous to the body than doing the washing up by hand over a properly fitted sink. Similarly, if you have a garden, balcony or veranda and the choice of drying clothes in a dryer or hanging your washing out on the line, we would definitely recommend the latter. Putting wet, heavy washing into a dryer (which is usually placed at floor-level) requires bending down and is a nuisance for the back. If, on the other hand, you go out into the sunshine and fresh air, reach up high to hang the washing and sing a song while doing so, the dreadful chore turns into a positive and joyful activity. Please yourself when you can.

Music and sound

In the same way that the Western world is being crippled by an overdose of food, it is also being force-fed with so-called conveniences such as television, radio, videos, records, tapes, CDs, telephones and faxes, and the flashing lights and noise of photocopiers and computers. All these machines are but extensions of our basic senses yet they often seem to take our lives over completely. The day is perhaps not far when some whizz-kid will invent a pocket-sized single piece of equipment to cover all these functions. Or even better, one day we might be able to implant a single chip into our brain which will take care of all our communication problems all at once.

Could there be a way to evolve to such super-capacity naturally? Who is to tell? In the meantime it is important not to let our conveniences take the upper hand. Again, eliminate the clutter of sound and glare. Noise and visual effects in a house can make or break the atmosphere. Modern equipment allows for fine-tuning ambient conditions, to answer different needs at different times. Constantly humming fridges, heaters, computers, etc. can drive the body crazy. The sounds in your home are as important as its ventilation, heating or lighting. In the morning, for example, when you are tidying up, you could put on some energetic music, follow the rules of proper postural conduct, and begin a ritual 'cleaning dance' as you are hoovering the floor or dusting the shelves. In this way, another horrid chore becomes fun and useful to your body. Late at night, when you feel romantic, don't wait for Christmas to light the candles and play soft music. Change and vary your habits – your body will begin to feel like it is on holiday all the time.

Lighting

In olden days the sun was worshipped as the most powerful source of energy. Even today, some remaining natural people in the more remote parts of South America and Africa pray to the sun and the moon for their daily needs. Here at home, health journals warn us of the danger of the sun, even accuse it of causing skin cancer. This is naturally very convenient for the creation of a whole range of new products and drugs which promise to 'protect' us from the evils of our mother star. But natural light is even more basic to life and health than air, food or sleep. Careful sun-focusing can improve your eyesight and mood and immensely regenerate your whole body. There is evidence that many syndromes, such as M.E. (myalgic ence-phalomyelitis), S.A.D. (seasonal affective disorder) and E.T.D. (emotional traumatic disorder) are caused, in part, by prolonged deprivation of light and clean air, by light and noise strain and other environmental factors.

It has always been taken for granted that air-conditioning and light bulbs are the same as fresh air and daylight, but they aren't the same at all, only poor substitutes for the real things. It also follows then that livestock, vegetables and plants grown in artificial light will lack the things that can only be found in real sunlight. We leave it to the scientists to work out what those ingredients are. We know that sunlight emits vital vitamins that are surely not contained in the radiation of an electric bulb.

To put it bluntly: if you cover a plant with a brown paper bag it will die. If you spend the winter months travelling before sunrise to work to spend the 'day' in an artificially lit, air-conditioned, centrally heated, synthetically carpeted office full of electronic and metallic equipment, only to return home in the dark to the waves emitted by your fridge, microwave and television set, then you may well become very ill indeed. If you are one of those poor people who doesn't get enough fresh air or daylight for months on end, try one of our enlightening moves for the eyes and face (page 70), to be performed outdoors when the sun comes up or just before it goes down whenever you get a chance to recharge your 'light and air battery'.

Weight loss

Y ou are not just what you eat, you are *how* and *why* you eat. You are also what you do, what you feel, what you think – in short, you are the sum total of all your senses and faculties. Once the problem of being overweight is detached from the food issue you are on your way to improving your shape. Losing weight is not about food, it is about the shape of your body. To take your mind off the food issue we have deliberately not given you any tantalizing photographs of delicious health recipes which would only make your mouth water. In this chapter we want to take the food issue off your mind altogether.

You are what, how and why you eat

The human body is, like any living thing, a vehicle for life. Food is only one of many energy sources, and satisfies only *one* of your many urges/senses. Regard your body for a moment as a hollow container through which many life-forces must circulate. Most life-forms need air, water, light, heat and energy, or they die. Some of us have forgotten about the basics and think we can live on the money that buys food, shelter and clothing. This is not enough. The immediate availability of food and consumer goods can soon turn you into a *bingeing shop-aholic*, and prey to food addiction, one of the many dangerous syndromatic epidemics of our age. An overfed, stagnant body that never moves much is going to become very unsatisfied. Not aware enough to identify the real cause of its discomfort, the food-addicted body is not sure why it is feeling unsatisfied and attempts to appease the vague sense of 'want', of feeling 'empty', by sneaking to the refrigerator, the chocolate box or the drinks cabinet for unnecessary, even harmful nourishment.

This cycle not only makes you fat, it also creates guilt, harms your self-esteem, can give you indigestion, piles, candida, colonitis, or stomach ulcers, make you obese, anorexic or bulimic, and even worse. You may think you are unable to change, but change is waiting at the end of the tunnel.

Change is life

A common misconception about the body is that it cannot change. The word 'cannot' does not exist in the body's movement vocabulary. By instinct, your friendly body always *tries* to feel better. Another delusion is that moving is tiring. On the contrary, good movement is reviving. Our approach to weight problems has always been that sensible physical expression is as essential to health as is the right kind of nutrition. So stop relating your weight problem to food, and prepare to be surprised.

The fat issue disclosed

There is nothing wrong with fat. Fat is not evil, it is not to be feared. Fat is comfortable, cuddly, and has many useful purposes. What is the function of fat? Fat serves to maintain body temperature and to provide padding, protection and support. A mother's belly stays fat after she gives birth because her baby needs this soft cushion to lie on while she is breastfeeding. That is, if the mother feeds her baby sitting on a chair. If she lies down on her side to feed, her belly will soon go away.

Fat also protects the precious marrow-containing bones. Fat is a safety device acquired by the body so that if you accidentally fall over you will not so easily break your bones. A fit muscle contracts (becomes hard and bouncy) on impact. The bone is then safe. If a muscle is so weak that it is not resilient and bouncy enough to protect the underlying bone from possible damage, then the body has to resort to the next best form of padding, which is fat tissue. The padding quality of fat also helps those who are less fit support their body parts when they are stuck in static positions for too long. People whose movement vocabulary is small, who don't use many muscles, often grow cushions of fat to be more comfortable.

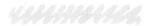

How do you get rid of fat?

Unused muscles are very easy beds for fat to grow on. Fat doesn't like change. Fat is harder than relaxed muscle. It's lazy, static and prefers not to be reminded of itself. Muscles can be toned up. Fat can't move, but it can disappear. The friendly body's first instinct is to be comfortable. It is therefore not going to keep a cumbersome lump of fat sitting on a spot where it would be in the way of a movement or even a position. As you vary your positions more your muscles tone up and the fat is no longer needed. It humbly retreats, to be absorbed and rejected by the body quite naturally.

How to be less hungry

Forget calories, nutritional values, additives, food with expiry dates, vitamins, minerals, pounds, kilos, inches or centimetres. Instead of food solutions to your weight problem, we suggest a lavish three-course meal: starter – relax in the 'baby pose' (page 54) and say hello to the fat on your stomach; main course – some well-done rolling moves; afters – the sweet feeling of permanent weight loss.

Rules for eating less

1. Empty your bowels before you eat

2. Stay well clear of meat
3. One or at most two meals a day
4. No drinking while eating

Empty your bowels before you eat

Sorry to begin so crudely, but the order of things demands that you empty your bowels before you eat.

If you have not been to the toilet today, don't eat breakfast, or even lunch, until you have. The body is a mere container for passing energy, thought and feeling. If you fill it up before it is emptied out, you will create blockages and traffic jams inside which will soon cause you discomfort. Fasting for a day or two has never done anyone any harm. It will clean you out, ready to start afresh. If you do decide to fast, drink plenty of water, not fruit juice; you don't need the acid or sugar.

Stay well clear of meat

Caution: The following story may contain text which might be offensive to some readers. We take the view, however, that although the story below may be a little unpalatable to read, it is a true account and an important lesson in health and safety.

Why we became vegetarian

A dance studio we worked at was situated in an inner London courtyard shared with the back entrance of a butcher's shop and the giant waste bins of a department store. Every morning a large van delivered huge carcasses of beef, halves of pigs, etc., which would then be weighed in the hot sunshine of the courtyard. The legs of beef that were being carried into the butcher's seemed much larger than the leg of any cow you might normally see in a field. The meat seemed swollen and very red. Flies were zooming from the bins to the meat, happily gorging themselves on fresh blood.

In the late afternoon, when all the butchers had gone home, stray dogs, cats and birds would negotiate any spare bones and leave their excretions behind. The odd derelict would come in drunk, looking for a corner to urinate in the now deserted yard.

It wasn't long after moving in that we called the health inspector, but it took a year to get the yard cleaned up and the butcher's scales moved *inside* their premises.

On Tuesday nights we would run a class called 'Big is Beautiful'. When we questioned our heavier clients about their diets our hunch was confirmed. They all turned out to be regular meat-eaters, some of them eating meat with every meal, full English breakfast included. Were there any weight-enhancing drugs and colouring agents in the meat? We became vegetarian just to be on the safe side.

The positive side of this nasty story is that we discovered a wealth of new tastes, spent a lot less time cooking, and we and our families have gained improved figures and better skin and teeth in the bargain. So if you are determined to lose weight fast, give up meat at once. After a few weeks, you won't even like it any more. Cooked meat will look to you like rubber and taste like cardboard. You don't need meat, you *are* meat. If you think it inconceivable to survive without meat, eat it only occasionally, but not more than twice a week.

One or at most two meals a day

An adult can live happily on one good meal a day. Drink plenty of water (at body temperature) before your meal to fill you up a little so you won't feel as hungry and won't want to eat too much, but eat yourself to the full. This meal is best taken in the late afternoon or early evening before relaxing or retiring, after the day's work has been done. 'Oh, but I would pass out if I didn't eat a little every few hours!' we hear you say. If you feel very hungry or tired during the day, eat a sandwich, but wait! Try this first and it will pick you up like a fresh breeze: find a place to lie down somewhere (every office should have one). Failing this, lie across your desk or on the carpeted floor for a few minutes. Stretch out fully, breathe deeply and relax. Sit up and drink plenty of fresh water. This will give you instant energy and you may not need that midday snack after all.

If you really must eat something, pretend you are a rabbit. Your teeth are made for chewing carrots, salads and all sorts of raw or almost raw vegetables, nuts and fruits. These contain tasty juices and fibre. You can eat as much as you want of these types of food on a piece of thinly buttered bread without gaining much weight at all. Look forward to your main meal by focusing on the texture, colour, aroma, composition, size and shape of what you are going to put inside your body. Integrate these qualities in your meal. Concentrate on how it feels to chew your food. Can you truly enjoy chewing a huge mouthful of food? Or is it more satisfying to savour an average bite?

No drinking while eating

A meal should be balanced in such a way that you don't need to 'drink' your food down. A bite of food should contain:

- enough raw, juicy vegetables or salad ingredients to moisten the mouth
- carbohydrates (bulk, like bread or potatoes) while chewing.

If you need to drink while you eat, it means that the composition of your meal is not right. Swallowing mushy, overcooked, dark brown food isn't appetizing and is bad for digestion and for the teeth, as it does away with the preliminary digestive process of chewing when saliva and its useful enzymes mixes with the food before it is piled up into the stomach. Rinse your mouth with water after eating (to clean your teeth) but don't, as a rule, drink during meals unless a special 'wine and dine' occasion demands the odd toast for good form.

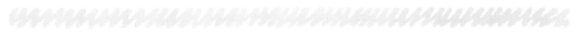

Weight loss in practice

In the next chapter you will learn the Kando moves that will reshape your body and systematically re-educate your daily movements. Follow the sections sequentially to begin with. Most moves are suitable for everyone unless marked as especially relevant to 'beginners', 'intermediate' or 'advanced' standards.

Don't hurry through the chapter. Learn about one or two new moves a day and incorporate them into your daily life. When you have reached the end of the chapter, don't put the book on a shelf to gather dust. Consult the daily, weekly and monthly progress chart on page 134. You may feel like a break from time to time but always return to your body's needs by treating it to this simple but most rejuvenating technique.

The Kando moves

Hips, bums, tums and thighs

Baby pose (Beginners)

The baby pose is one of the most comfortable positions for easing indigestion or combating fatigue or distress. It helps you to pass wind and to stimulate bowel motion.

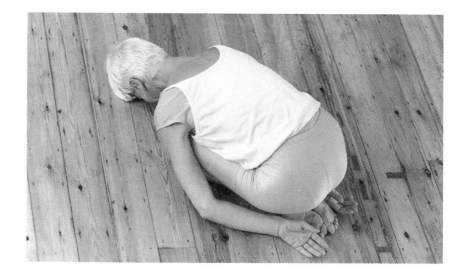

Figure 10: Baby pose

1. Kneel down on a soft mat, sitting on your heels.
2. Let your head sink down toward the floor, bringing your whole body forward until it is supported and relaxed.
3. Your arms should also rest on the floor, down by your sides, with your shoulders rotating inwards, palms up as shown (Figure 10).
4. Rest your head on one side, on your cheek or one ear if you can. If it won't reach that far, just let your head hang loose and relax your neck and shoulders.
5. Relax your whole body and breathe quietly.
6. Close your eyes.
7. Enjoy it.

Breakfast move: Licking the plate (Intermediate)

1. Take up the 'baby pose' and stretch your arms out far over your head on the floor (Figure 11a). Relax.
2. On an in-breath, keep your hands where they are and glide your forehead along the floor, all the way to the prone position as shown in Figure 11b. Breathe out and rest.
3. On the next in-breath, lift your torso off the ground.
4. While it is lifted, perform a slow head roll in each direction (Figure 11c).
5. Come to rest again with one cheek on the floor. Take a deep breath, ready for the return journey.
6. Lifting your bottom, but keeping your forehead near the floor, return to the baby pose.

For fat legs and ankles (water retention)

1. Whenever you get an opportunity, take your socks and shoes off and put your feet higher than chest-level (above your heart) to alleviate the downward pressure of gravity.
2. Massage your feet and legs.
3. Lie back with your legs high up in the air and kick vigorously upwards towards the ceiling.
4. Massage and scratch the area behind your knees with your knuckles. This prevents varicose veins, moves along stagnant fat dimples (cellulite), loosens your knee joints and improves articulation in your whole leg.

*Figure 11: Licking
the plate*

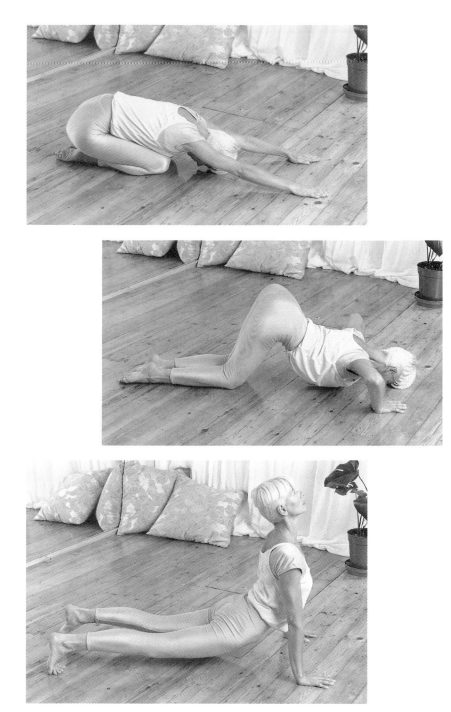

Are you chairbound?

One of the main causes of back pain and fat hips, bums, tums and thighs is that people sit on chairs too much. Most of our waking hours is spent sitting – at breakfast, on the bus, in the car, at work, at lunch, at the dinner table, in the toilet, in fact if we are not either walking or sleeping we are probably sitting. Holding a position is the most tiring form of physical activity. It takes more energy and effort to stand absolutely still for ten minutes than to run around the block. To see if your hamstrings (the muscle group behind the knees) have become shortened by too much sitting, do the following short experiment:

1. Lie on your back on a bed or on the floor.
2. Now lift your knees up towards your chest and try to stretch your legs so they are at right angles to the bed or floor.

Note: Make sure your whole spine, from the back of your head down to your coccyx (the lowest bone in the spine) remains flat on the floor, otherwise you will be cheating.

What shape is your body making? Is it dangerously looking like b) in Figure 12? If this is the case and you cannot stretch your legs fully, don't panic, short hamstrings can stretch, even in maturity and old age.

Figure 12:
a) supple;
b) chairbound

3. Gently kick your legs upwards towards the ceiling to stretch your hamstrings.

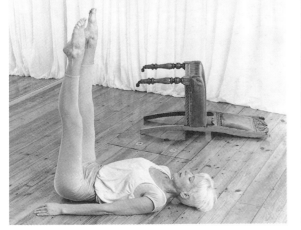
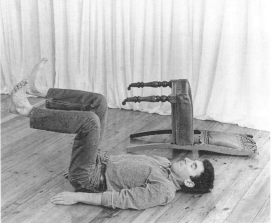

*Figure 13: The
sitting bones:
a) rock to left;
b) centre;
c) rock to right*

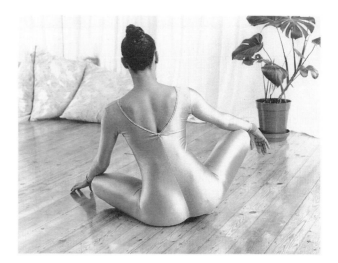

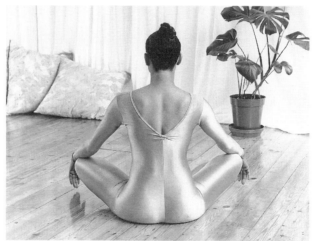

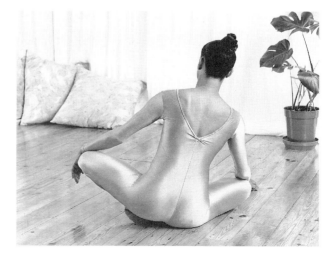

4. Sit up with your legs as straight as possible in front of you and relax the area behind your knees. Massage behind your knees and breathe out deeply.

Feeling the sitting bones

Sitting on the floor gives full rest to your feet, ankles and knees. When your legs are supported horizontally, circulation is more efficient and less demanding on your heart. The sitting bones are the two lowest protrusions of your pelvic bone. They can be felt when you sit on the floor, or on a hard chair, and rock from side to side. The sitting bones are your own, built-in seat.

Like the legs of a two-legged stool, your sitting bones support the upper half of your body. Additional support comes from your legs to help you keep your trunk balanced when sitting.

Sitting on your own built-in seat

On the floor you discover the furniture built into your own body millions of years ago. The biggest advantage of not using a chair is that sitting may be varied. You have many options for changing position, giving many more different muscles a share in the

Figure 14: Your built-in seat

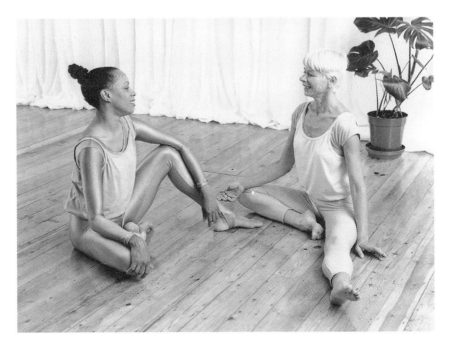

action – spreading the load, as it were. You will find that you can apply yourself to a task done while sitting on the floor for much longer, that you will get less tired in the process and become more flexible, slimmer and more efficient in the bargain.

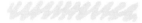

Hips, bums and tums

Now try some typical hip, bum and tum games, which you can do either alone or with a few friends instead of having tea and biscuits.

Bum racing (for any number of players)

1. Sit up straight with your legs straight out in front of you. Keep your pelvis erect and your spine straight; relax your shoulders.
2. On the word 'Go!' race across the room and back again on your bum (the sitting bones). The first person back is the winner. Don't cheat and use your hands. They should stay off the floor throughout.

Wobble, wobble, all fall down

1. Sit on the floor with enough room on either side to extend your arms out fully.
2. Bring your arms down and begin to sway from side to side, lifting one bum cheek up, then the other until you almost lose your balance. Your hands may be used for support (Figure 15a).
3. Continue the rocking motion while at the same time lowering your back towards the floor until you eventually end up flat on your back, but still rolling from side to side (Figure 15b).
4. The movement may be extended to a half roll and backward kick as shown in Figure 15c.

Spinning top

1. Kneel on the floor and shift your bum to the right so that your right hip is supporting your weight.
2. Bring your knees up and over to your left side to reverse the position.
3. Now lift your bum and sit on your right side again.

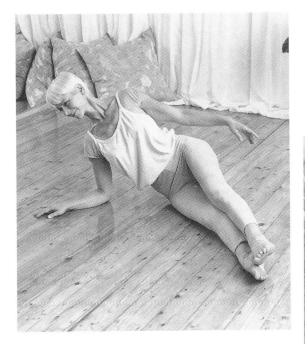

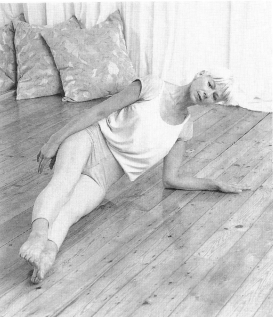

Figure 15:
Wobble, wobble
with half roll and
backward kick

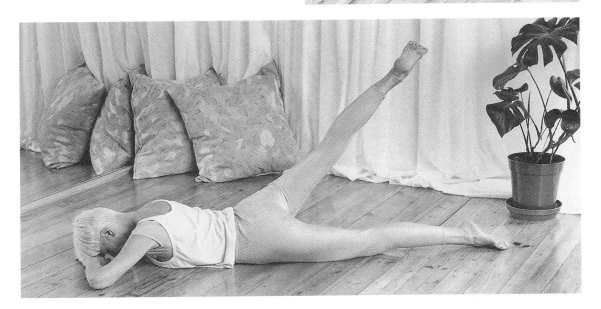

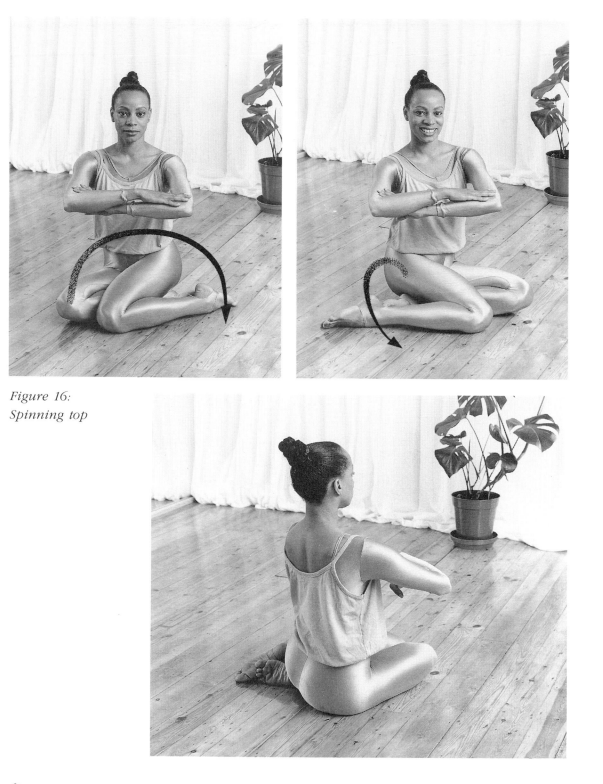

Figure 16:
Spinning top

4. Repeat from 2, picking up your knees and bringing them over to the left. Lift your seat over your feet and carry on like this to make continuous circles travelling around the room.

Note: You may use your hands at first. Try to keep your spine vertical throughout. Take power from your thighs and stomach (relax those shoulders!). The spinning top strengthens your knees and tones your stomach, waist, thigh and back muscles all at once. Eventually, when you are stronger, you should be able to do it without your hands and twirl around the room. It will massage all superfluous lumps of fat away and tone your muscles. When you are done, you can dig into a nutritious meal without the worry of unwanted padding.

As you get used to eating less, drinking more water and moving better, your stomach will shrink and your persistent hunger diminishes. A fat person's hunger is merely the body's expression of discomfort or emotional dissatisfaction. Whenever you feel tired and listless, in the mood for bingeing, your body is showing a *genuine need* which will never be satisfied with food. For an overfed body, movement and breathing are much more gratifying than eating.

From now on, all moves and games given in the technique are going to reduce unwanted fat, as they are designed to make you feel and move better. But rather than suffering the pains of cruel diets and exhausting exercise, get into the habit of sitting on the floor more often and varying your position in the many ways offered here. This will force the fat off your bum, hips and thighs as your underlying bone structure feels that it wants to be held in balance by its own healthy muscles rather than be supported by insensitive and cumbersome lumps of fat squashed between your body and an armchair.

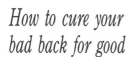

Back, neck, shoulders and face

How to cure your bad back for good

How many times have you read statistics about the number of working hours lost through back injuries? In fact, it is rare for anyone over the age of 35 not to have had any backache complaints. Is your back killing you again? We address the cause of your trouble by instantly releasing pain through relaxation, passive articulation (gentle moves) and massage. The following four moves are variations on the 'baby pose' given on page 54. You didn't really think the baby was going to lie still all night, did you?

Figure 17: Baby pose with turn-out

Figure 18: Baby pose with one leg outstretched

Baby pose with turn-out

Assume the baby pose and then open your knees and allow your body weight to drop between them. This gives more of a turn-out in your groin and gets you even closer to mother gravity.

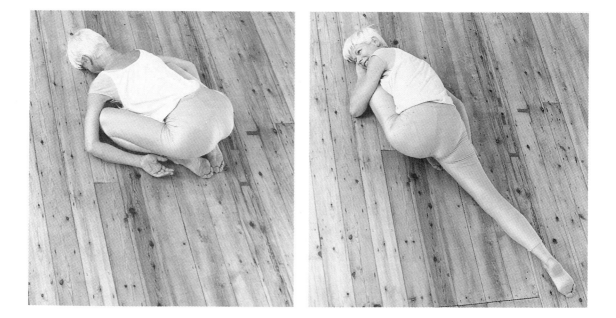

Baby pose with one leg outstretched

In this variation of the baby pose you stretch one leg.

Baby pose with one leg bent to the side

One last, most 'comfy' baby pose, if you can get down to it. Bring your bent knee out to the side to allow your weight to sink much deeper into the floor. This relaxes your body even further.

Figure 19: Baby pose with one leg bent to the side

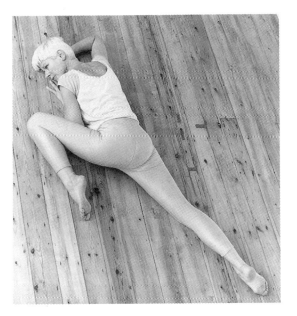

Try the above two poses on the other side.

Now that your spine is fully relaxed, we may begin improving its shape.

Like a bead necklace or a chain, your spine is made up of loose vertebrae and is actually mobile. All you need to do to begin loosening your spine is to lie down on the floor, on your back.

Caution: For people with chronic back pain, scoliosis (sideways spinal curve) or sclerosis (hardening of tissues), this position may, at first, feel slightly uncomfortable and should not be attempted without support. If you are not used to lying on the floor comfortably, begin by supporting the parts that are too stiff (behind your knees, waist and neck areas) with little cushions, mats or bolsters. As time goes on and you begin to straighten out a little and grow, you can gradually lessen the size of the supports until eventually your skeleton will lie as flat as a pancake and feel comfortable. Take it step by step and you won't suffer.

Correct neck alignment (Advanced)

1. Place a low stool plus some soft mats by the end of your bed to construct a surface that will allow your neck to lie in its proper place.

Note: The aim is to place the back of your neck *in line with your spinal column*. The back of your skull is now receding, instead of lying on a lump, bump or hump where a pillow would normally be. Breathing is thereby also improved as the air passages are more open in this way. Don't forget to keep your chin down and lengthen the back of your neck.

Figure 20: Correct neck alignment

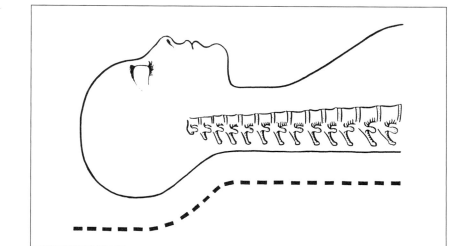

Lengthening the torso (Beginners)

1. Lie on the floor on your back. Put your hands on your waist, at the top of your hip bones.
2. Now start 'walking' with your shoulder blades away from your waist. It is possible in this way to keep your buttocks and legs in one place while your upper back moves away, towards your head. This stretches your spine and frees downward pressure on it.

Horizontal twist (Beginners)

This move is particularly good for releasing pressure on the sciatic nerve.

1. Lie on your back and pull your knees high up towards your chest. Your arms should be stretched out away from you on the floor at shoulder height. Breathe in deeply.
2. On an out-breath, bring both knees together down towards the floor beside you on your right.
3. Turn your head to the left so that your left cheek is resting on the floor.
4. Relax all the muscles in your body and stay there for a while, breathing deep down into your abdomen.
5. Take another deep in-breath and reverse the position, this time picking up your knees and bringing them down on your left side beside you and turning your head towards the right. Rest.

Figure 21:
Horizontal twist

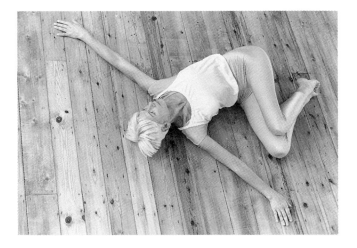

Ironing out your spine (Intermediate)

This move is nice to do every morning to get your body going at full gear. It is a yoga move called the Plough.

1. Lie down on your back.
2. Bring your knees high up above your chest.
3. With the help of your hands pushing behind your waist, push yourself up and over until your feet touch the ground behind your head.

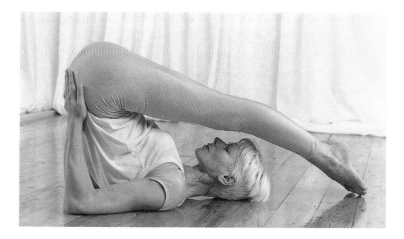

Shoulder stand (Advanced Only)

Caution: Do not stay in a shoulder stand unless you are very fit. The weight of your legs presses down exactly on the sensitive area of the lower back, where nerves may be trapped.

Figure 23:
Shoulder stand
(only for the fit)

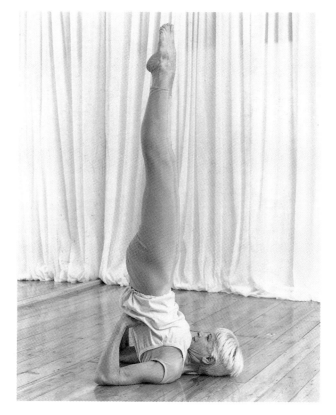

4. Take a few breaths while still in position 3 of Ironing out your spine (above). Relax your legs, shoulders and neck.

So far so good, but you are not finished yet. How do you come back? This is the most important part of the move, so pay careful attention:

5. Slowly bring your spine back to the floor, starting at the upper vertebrae, one bone at a time until your whole spine is flat on the floor again.

Note: *Don't* tense your shoulders and let your body fall back to the floor like a stiff banana, letting your neck and head come off the floor. Instead, bring your spine and legs down while leaving your upper back, shoulders, *neck and head relaxed* on the floor. This is not easy at first, but it will make your stomach and thigh muscles work harder and really give your upper back and neck a jolly good ironing out.

Figure 24: Coming back from the Plough: a) incorrect; b) correct

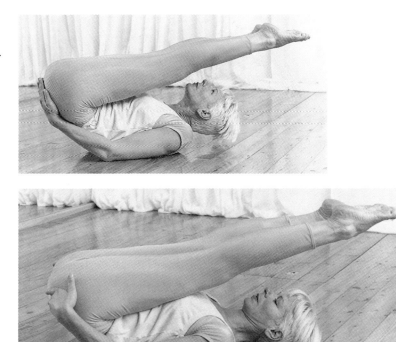

For the eyes
and face

Safe sun-focusing

1. Stand outside, somewhere in a field or garden, and face the pale sun.
2. Close your eyes and put the palm of your right hand over your right eye.
3. Peer through the gaps between your fingers. Find the sun and, with your right eye only, focus upon it. Keep looking at the sun until it stops wobbling around like a yo-yo and becomes still, a perfectly clean, clear white disc.
4. At this moment, breathe in as deep as you can and absorb the white sunlight deep down into your body, all the way to your toes. Your solar plexus will make a jump and you should feel a sudden feeling of ecstasy – a 'sungasm'.
5. Now cover both eyes and relax them. The imprint you see on your retina is not really there; ignore it and try to see pure, clean darkness.
6. Take a few deep breaths before repeating from 3 above with your left eye.
7. If you feel up to it, repeat again with both eyes. If not, do this focusing again in a few days' time. Eventually you will be able to achieve 'sungasm' – without having to put your palms over your eyes – anytime you feel like it. To begin with, however, don't do it more than once a week.

Note: Your eyes might want to cry the first time you try a 'sungasm'. Don't resist. Don't rub your eyes violently with your fists, either, as this stretches your skin and creates wrinkles. Instead, just allow a few tears to cleanse your eyes from the inside and drain out all your worries.

Pirouette with the sun (Intermediate)

1. Again stand outside in the pale or orange sunshine.
2. Now slowly turn on the spot without losing sight of the sun.

Note: This rotation forces your neck, upper back and shoulders to move in a gradual backward-bending position, loosening this top part of your spine. The object is to keep your eyes on the sun and not to lose it. Good luck and have fun with it.

Realignment

When your body is horizontal, as when you are lying on the floor, the force of gravity is distributed equally – each bone carries only its own weight.

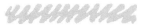

Rolling

In the following rolls gravity can be used to your body's advantage to help it find its centre and realign its bones in a more balanced way.

Quarter rolls with balance and flop

1. Lie on the floor on your back with your feet together. Your legs should be straight out and your arms raised, hands resting on the floor above your head.
2. Take a quarter roll to the right so you are lying on your right side. Now make your body very stiff. Tighten your buttocks and lengthen your whole spine outward, stretching your hands out and stiffening up to find your line of balance, which should be resting on your right leg, hip, side, armpit and arm. Your head is resting on your right arm. Now breathe in and *stay balanced* in this position.
3. Suddenly let your body flop onto its front, letting go of all tension on an out-breath.
4. Roll on a quarter turn onto your *left* side and again become stiff as a plank and find your balance.
5. On a sudden out-breath, which could even be accompanied by a noise of relief, let go of all tension and *flop* over to end up where you started, lying on your back.

Note: The whole sequence is just a roll, but every time you are lying on your side you should be outstretched and balanced, every time you are prone or supine (facing the floor or the ceiling), your body is relaxed and floppy. Note how your breathing accompanies the two opposing dynamic qualities of the move: inhale before balance, exhale to flop into relaxation.

Quarter rolls with kicks (Intermediate)

This is a progression of the previous move. In each new quarter roll, kick one leg up into the air. Again, the object of the game is to find balance when lying on your side and to check that your alignment is correct while in the prone and supine positions.

Figure 25: Quarter rolls with kicks

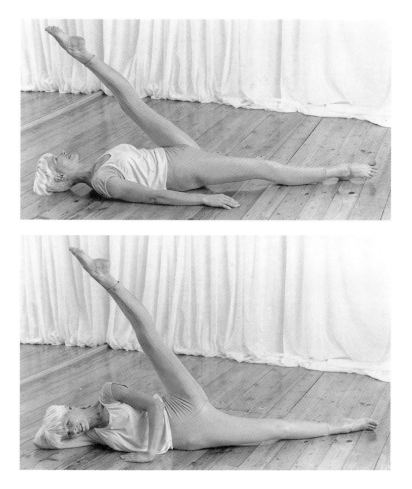

Quarter rolls with body curve (Advanced)

Roll again, slowly through each direction, but this time lift both legs and both arms up each time you change position.

Continuous rolling (Beginners)

Even before any of the above moves are well mastered, you will enjoy just rolling on the floor with your arms above your head. This releases tension and realigns your body at the same time. People often get the giggles when they roll; it seems to be one of the most alleviating moves we have come across. Although we introduced rolling with alignment and tension-relief in mind, another benefit is that regular rolling also reduces unwanted bellies and 'spare tyres'.

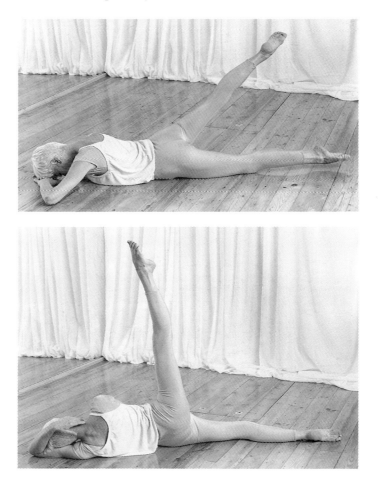

Stance and balance

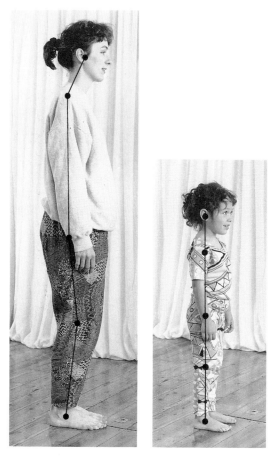

Figure 26: Posture:
a) adult; b) child

Balance requires that body parts are placed in equilibrium in relation to their centre of gravity. The human condition of living upright is like being a tree without roots, or a bird without wings. The spine had to develop compensating curves in order to absorb shock and to give enough counter-balance for the body weight pushing down on a drastically reduced base area. But how deep are curves in the spine meant to be? Do we have to wait for an acute attack of migraine, sciatica or a slipped disc to find out our spine curves too much? Look at a three-year-old's spine: you'll see that the curves are not at all the same as the curves in an adult spine. Young children's heads are so large and heavy in proportion to their bodies that if they were to hold their heads the way adults do, in front of their bodies, they would simply fall over.

Looking at Figure 26, observe the line of gravity passing through the skeleton. The other difference between an adult's and a child's posture is that children tend to absorb shock in their feet and legs, whereas adults take most weight in the spinal column, hence the deeper spinal curves that often cause so much pain. However these can be straightened out (see 'Back, Neck, Shoulders and Face', beginning on page 64).

A standing posture has to be built from the ground up. The problem with many adults today is that their feet are not really in good enough shape to bear the weight of the body in a balanced way. Instead, feet are often squashed in narrow, pointed shoes which prevent them from supporting the body's weight efficiently. So lesson number one in postural realignment is always to have a thorough look at your feet first.

Building the foundations – the feet

Now that your spine is as long as it can be, let us see if we can rebuild your body from its base, starting at your feet. It is not easy to support a tall, upright thing like a human body on a pair of feet that have lost the full use of their toes and lost the bounce in their arches. To explain this further, look at your foot as if it were the roots of a tall tree. The narrower and smaller the roots are, the more easily the tree will fall over or be uprooted by a heavy storm. Full potential balance and support in the foot is the very first thing to consider when you are dealing with rebalancing your body to move well. Like a kitten's paw, your foot is made for balance and jumping.

Foot alignment

Figure 27: Top side of the foot (seen from above)

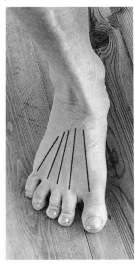

Take your shoes and socks off for a moment and take a look at your feet. You will see that the main body of your foot is, like your hands, made up of a number of fan-shaped bones which spread outwards towards your toes. The shape of these bones indicates where your toes should be aligned, namely as a continuation of the fan-shaped bones.

Now look at your toes and see how much you can move them outwards and whether their shape matches the fan-shaped bones to which they are attached. If your toes won't move outward much at all, you need to reawaken them so that once again they will be in a position to share the weight-bearing when you are standing, walking, jumping and running. The foot is designed to bear weight equally on the two pads of each toe, the two pads under your forefoot and the one large pad under your heel.

The areas of the sole of the foot that don't touch the ground form your feet's *arches*. Each arch is cleverly constructed to take pressure in two directions at once. First there is a long arch going

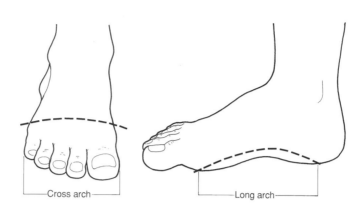

Figure 28: a) the long arch; b) the cross arch of the foot

Cross arch

Long arch

from the ball of your foot towards your heels. When you stand correctly, this arch should rise like a bridge. The second arch goes across the width of your forefoot, as shown in Figure 28b.

Together these arches form a veritable *spring plank* and are capable of absorbing shock from jumps even without your having to bend your knees at all. To test this out for yourself:

Bouncing

1. Place your feet close together.
2. Bounce gently up and down without bending your knees. The movement in your ankle joints makes you bounce but the landing impact is absorbed by your feet only.

What is shown here is that there is plenty of inherent bounce in the foot and toes even before resorting to the knee, let alone the spine, for further shock absorption. Once your feet are firmly on the ground and efficiently sharing your body weight, your movements can become more balanced, easier, freer and stronger.

Building a balanced posture

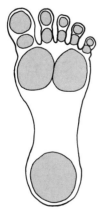

Figure 29: A healthy human footprint

Now that you have a strong, wide base to stand on and you know where all the bits should go in relation to gravity and with regard to the structure of your body itself, it should be easy to build up a near-perfect standing posture which will take the least effort to hold and look most attractive.

1. Stand with your feet shoulder- or hip-width apart, whichever is the widest, taking care that your toes are spread and your arches lifted.
2. Relax your knees (don't lock them) and keep your pelvis straight (tuck it under if you have a protruding bum and tummy).
3. On an in-breath, lift your ribcage.
4. Breathe out and relax your shoulders.

Shoulder placement

Aim to keep your arms at your sides, rather than hanging in front like a monkey. But *never pull your shoulders back* as this will

Figure 30:
Shoulder placement:
a) incorrect;
b) corrective move;
c) improved
placement

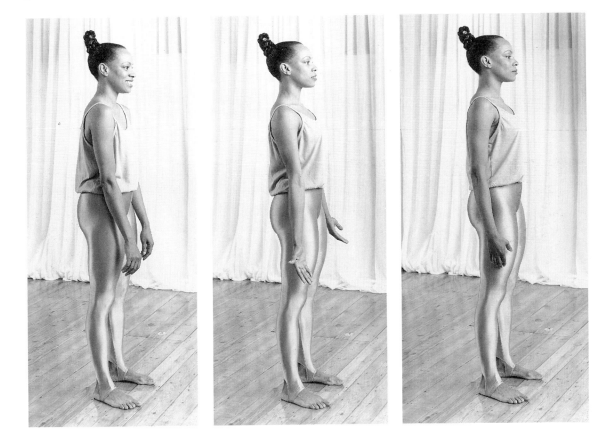

only distort your posture, make you look like an uptight sergeant major, and make your upper back even weaker and narrower. If your arms don't naturally fall by your sides, rotate the palms of your hands forwards and outwards to *turn out* your shoulder joint. This action lengthens the muscles between your chest and shoulders. It opens your wings.

Note: When you have reached position b), hold the turn-out in your shoulders but relax your forearms. The palms of your hands will now naturally rotate back towards the front, to give you the correct position.

Neck and head placement

We continue building up your skeleton:

1. Centre your neck at the top of your spine. Pretend you are a kitten being picked up by the back of the neck. Pull the back of your neck back and up, yet *keep your chin down*.
2. Look up slightly, towards an imaginary horizon.
3. Your head, which is resting on the atlas (the top vertebra in the spinal column, situated somewhere between your ears) is now able to balance with a minimum of effort. You should be feeling as if your crown were pulling you up.

Note: In this correct position, your eyes should not be able to see any part of your body. If you can see your knees, thighs or bust, it means you are leaning forward. Don't pull your shoulders back, either. Keep your upper back wide by imagining that your shoulders are moving out sideways and down, then gently try the next spinal twists.

Standing spinal twists

1. Stand with feet apart, knees relaxed, your arms hanging loosely by your sides.
2. Look back and to the right as far as you can, while keeping your feet, knees and hips firmly facing front.
3. Come back to face front and repeat to the left.
4. Carry on twisting to the right and left alternately, keeping your

Figure 31: Standing spinal twists

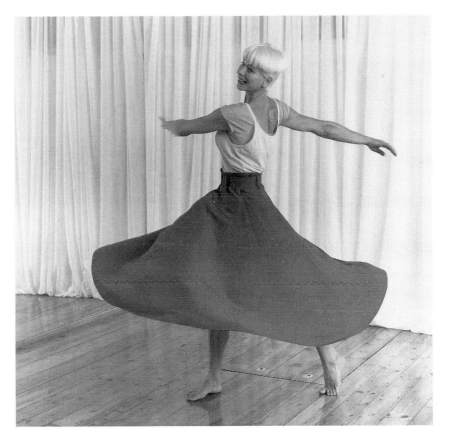

arms limp, while increasing momentum as you proceed – not necessarily making faster twists but looser and larger ones, and looking further behind you each time until you have done about twelve to sixteen twists, then decrease momentum to come back to standing facing front.

Note: How far can you see behind you? The action is initiated by your full peripheral vision. This full spinal twist works wonders on stiff backs, shoulders and necks.

Turning on the spot

Turning is for the body like winding or unwinding a spring. It works to wind you up when you are tired or wind you down when you are too tense. In both cases, turning is one of the most therapeutic moves at our body's disposal and should be used almost on a daily basis, just to shake out a lot of accumulated tension and aggravation we can well do without, or to summon up courage and strength for new challenges ahead. As mentioned earlier, balance is heavily reliant on vision. In the beginning, therefore, use your eyes to *spot* direction, which helps you keep your balance while turning. When you are doing a full clockwise turn, you will be facing the front, the right, the back and the left successively. Use your eyes to locate a spot to focus on in each direction.

1. *Beginners*: With both feet on the floor, face the front, the right, the back and the left respectively to finish again facing the front.
2. Start as for 1. Then take little jumps on both feet as you turn in each direction.
3. *Intermediate*: Turn as for 1, but stand on one foot only.
4. As for 1; this time jumping round on two feet.
5. *Advanced*: Jump on one foot only through all directions.

Repeat the moves going anti-clockwise, towards the *left*, changing legs where appropriate.

Note: Make sure you land in each predetermined direction by focusing with your eyes.

Dervish turn (Intermediate)

1. Stand on your right foot with your left foot just behind it resting on its ball. Hold your arms out at shoulder height; your right palm should be facing down, your left palm facing up. Lift your head and look up at the ceiling.
2. A slight weight transference from your right foot to the ball of your left foot makes you turn your body around bit by bit clockwise.
3. Repeat the ball, step, ball, step action with your feet, gradually increasing the momentum of your turn.

Note: Your eyes should not be bothered by the blur of the room swishing past. Focus on a spot above your head on the ceiling with your eyes for stability while your body is spinning round its own line of gravity. Real dervishes can do this continuous turn for hours on end as a form of meditation. For our purposes, don't continue if you get too dizzy – but do allow a little dizziness to occur. Then repeat immediately on the other side to 'unwind' you back to normal.

The degree to which each joint allows for free, easy movement is surprisingly greater than you ever thought possible. Even in an old and misused body, the urge to move well is inherent. As long as you approach the matter gently and in a physically-friendly way, your body will be only too pleased to give you remarkable results, as you will discover when you do the following articulation moves.

Articulation – lying down

We'll start at the very extremity of your body, your toes.

Toe-pulling

1. Sitting on the floor, take hold of the little toe of your right foot with both hands.
3. Gently pull and turn the toe around. You might hear a little cracking noise in one of its little joints – this is fine. It's your little toe's way of saying hello.
4. Repeat with the next toe until it makes itself heard just once.
5. Move on to the next toe and so on until you have done all the toes on your right foot.
6. Stretch your legs out, lie down for a few seconds and begin again with your left foot.

Note: In older people the big toe won't budge much, but try to lengthen it and get it to move as much as possible towards the inside of your foot.

Moving your ankles

1. Sit on the floor with your feet in front of you. Try to keep your legs straight if you can. If you can't, just bend your knees a little, propping up your back.
2. Flex and point your feet eight or more times until your ankles stop 'singing' and you are sure that they move fully.
3. Now rotate your ankles several times outward, away from each other.
4. Now rotate them inward, towards each other. Listen out for some more noises.

Moving your knees

The knee joint needs to be kept loose, otherwise no amount of bending, squatting or comfortable sitting on the floor will be possible. Also, if your knees are stiff they become weak and hamper walking, running and jumping. If you have weak knees you should definitely do the following gentle knee movements.

1. Lie down on your back, knees bent, feet on the floor.
2. Take your right knee in your hands (but leave your head comfortably on the floor) and put your left palm on your right knee-cap.
3. Now, while your hand is 'listening' to your knee, gently bend and stretch your leg. Do you hear any noises? Does your hand feel any cracking or squeaking?
4. Now hold the knee in one place and circle your foot round and round in both directions.
5. Carry on articulating your knee until the noise stops.
6. Stretch your leg out fully, rest and change legs.
7. Repeat with your other knee.

Loosening your knees

1. Lying on the floor, kick both legs up towards the ceiling as if trying to throw off your shoes. This will really loosen your knee joints. Accept any little cracking noises as happy awakening songs.
2. Bring your legs down on the floor and shake them loose before doing the following sitting sequences, which will further stretch and bend your knees to their full range.

Moving your legs

The hip joints connect the legs to the trunk. They are the largest and the most weight-bearing joints in the body, after the ankle and knee joints, as they support the pelvis, the trunk, shoulders, arms and head, in short everything above the legs. Much trouble later in life can be averted now by keeping this major joint strong and mobile. A last-resort hip operation is like underpinning the subsiding second floor of your body's edifice. Don't let it come to that if you can help it now! The hip joint's most frequent move is the forward motion. But often, through restricted living habits, this movement has been reduced to nothing. We can increase its range by stretching the hamstrings.

Stretching your hamstrings (Beginners)

The hamstrings, the bundle of muscles behind your knees, are shortened in most 'normal' adults due to a lack of mobility and to sitting too much. Can you touch the floor while standing with your knees straight? Hands flat on the floor? Standing on the tip of your toes? If not, you need to stretch your hamstrings. Try this easy one first.

1. Sit on the floor with your bum against a wall. Pull up your ribcage to a balanced sitting posture, but leave your shoulders relaxed. Your whole spine and the back of your head should be touching the wall behind you.
2. Bend forward. Pretend to go to sleep on your knees, relax and breathe deeply into the stretching sensation. Breathing and letting go will gradually stretch your hamstrings for you. You don't have to 'do' anything, just let it happen, all by itself. Let go and take your time over it. You could, for example, go through your mail in this position.

Note: Rub the area behind your knees with your knuckles to help move along accumulated stiffness.

Next, we introduce movements that are less frequently used in normal adult behaviour: the turn-out, the turn-in, and backward and sideways articulation of the hip joint.

Figure 32: Turn-out: a) sit on the floor or in the bath facing the side with one knee on the floor, the other supporting your elbow; b) one knee on the floor, your other leg straight; c) the half lotus; d) full lotus

Turn-out

Tightness in the hip joint is strongest in Western women who have, for ages, followed a fashion that told them to keep their legs crossed and squeezed together. This centuries-old habit has created what is now termed *groin tension*, the most tense area in the body after the neck and shoulder region. It is in the rarely

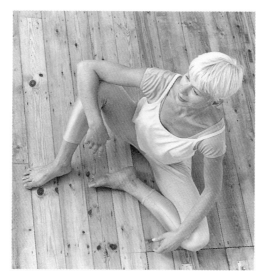

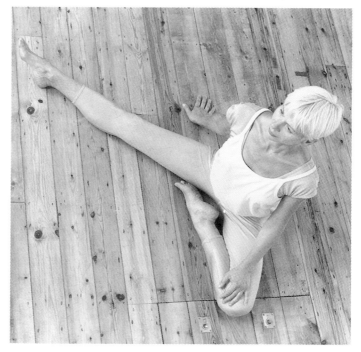

used outward and backward directions that the hip joint needs re-articulating most. It won't hurt a bit if you do some of these in the bath (facing the side of the bath for more room) when your body is soft and warm. The object in all examples is to allow your knees to drop down deeper towards the floor.

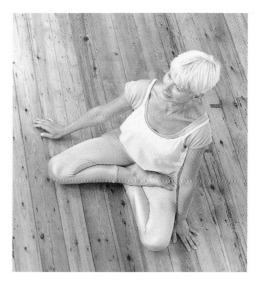

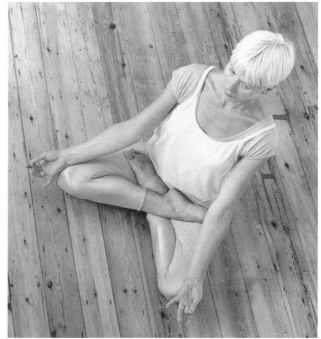

Figure 33: One-legged turn-in:
a) holding your foot
with your hand;
b) with strap

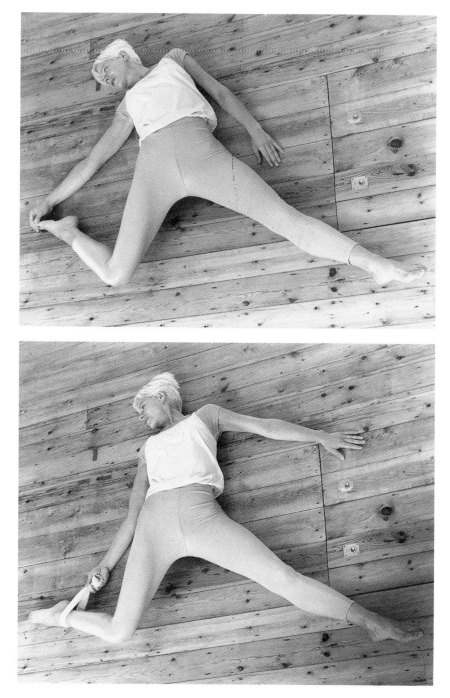

One-legged turn-in (Beginners)

Turning the leg inwards is the opposite of a turn-out and requires more space. It cannot be done in the bath unless you have a *big* one.

1. Lie down on your back with your left leg straight and your right leg turned in and bent by your side.
2. Hold your right foot with your right hand and gently pull it towards you. If you can't reach it, hold a canvas strap hooked around your ankle to help you.
3. Allow your right knee to drop slowly but surely closer towards the floor with each deep out-breath.

Note: There will, of course, be a pulling sensation along the front part of your groin, your thigh, perhaps even in the ligaments on the front of your right knee. This is exactly what you are aiming for. When the feeling becomes quite strong, massage the area. Imagine that your hand is talking to your right groin, thigh and knee and saying: 'It's all right folks, don't worry, just let go.'

Turn-out and turn-in

The following move gives each leg a different action, combining the turn-out and turn-in. Get into the position slowly and remember to aim for lowering your knees towards the floor.

Figure 34: Turn-out and turn-in

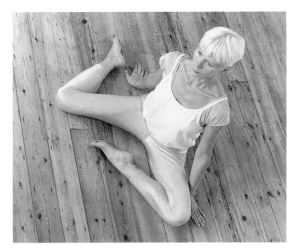

Don't forget to do it both sides.

A lack of mobility in the legs adds to groin tension. This is often worse for high-heel wearers, as their 'Y' ligaments (the strong bands that attach the leg to the front of the hip) are shortened, as explained earlier. You need the full use of this backward range for running and leaping, or if you are not that energetically inclined, just for relaxing gently and feeling energy flowing through a newly discovered part of your body. Lengthening the front of your thigh and hip improves your balance and posture tremendously and, by correcting the position of the pelvis, will also reduce your tummy and bum, remember?

Sitting on your heels and resting back in the bath (Beginners)

1. Kneel on both knees, on a soft bath mat if necessary.
2. Sit on your heels.
3. Now let your body lean backwards until you reach the back of the bath. Help with your arms and hands where necessary.

Note: Try to point your feet so that your instep is on the floor. If you get foot cramp, flex and massage the sole of your foot and try again.

Figure 35: Sitting on your heels (shown without bath)

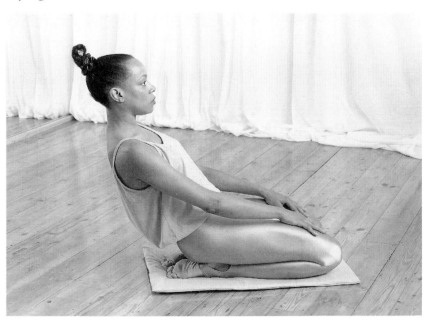

Folding your legs under (Advanced)

You are on the floor on a soft mat instead of in the bath.

1. Repeat 1 to 3 of the previous move.
2. Lower your upper body further until your head, neck and shoulders are on the floor (Figure 36a). 'Help! This feels dodgy . . .' Don't worry.
3. Drop your seat between your feet (Figure 36b). You are an omelette, flat and relaxed.
4. Breathe deeply and massage the front part of your upper leg and hip with a sympathetic hand while working out how on earth you are going to get out of this predicament.

Figure 36: Folding your legs under

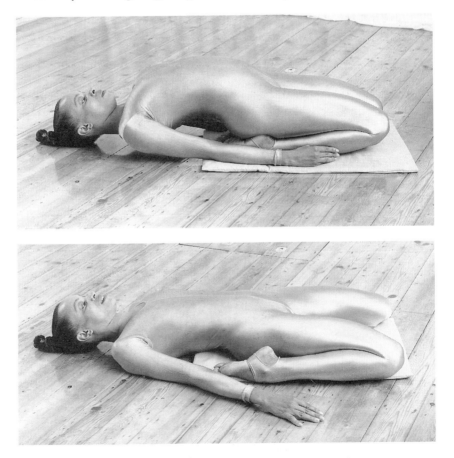

Note: *Do not* try to come up head first unless you have a strong back and strong stomach muscles. Instead, roll gently onto your stomach and get up from there.

Circling your legs (Beginners)

Circling your leg, or full articulation in the hip joint, involves movement in many directions.

1. Lie on your back on the floor with your feet together.
2. Pull up your *left* knee high up towards your chest as far as it can go and hold it with both hands. Your lower leg should be bent but relaxed.
3. Drop your knee towards the floor beside you.
4. Bring it up again.
5. Drop your knee across your body moving it gently towards your right side.
6. Continue to make slow knee circles: out, up, in, across your chest, two or three times. The movement may become larger and involve your pelvis as well. See how you go.
7. When you've finished, swap sides to repeat leg circling with your right leg.

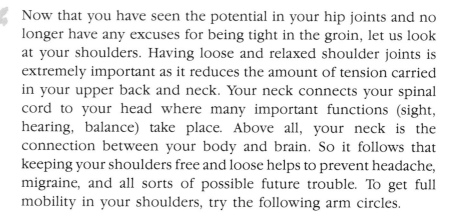

Flexibility in your shoulder joints

Now that you have seen the potential in your hip joints and no longer have any excuses for being tight in the groin, let us look at your shoulders. Having loose and relaxed shoulder joints is extremely important as it reduces the amount of tension carried in your upper back and neck. Your neck connects your spinal cord to your head where many important functions (sight, hearing, balance) take place. Above all, your neck is the connection between your body and brain. So it follows that keeping your shoulders free and loose helps to prevent headache, migraine, and all sorts of possible future trouble. To get full mobility in your shoulders, try the following arm circles.

Arm circling on the floor (Beginners)

1. Lie on your back and drop your knees to the left. Then straighten your legs so that they are at right angles to your body. Your arms should rest outwards on the floor at shoulder height. Relax but try to keep both shoulders on the floor (Figure 37a).
2. Now look at your right hand and follow it with your eyes as it begins to circle: passing over your legs and across your face, way up above your head and diagonally up and outwards.

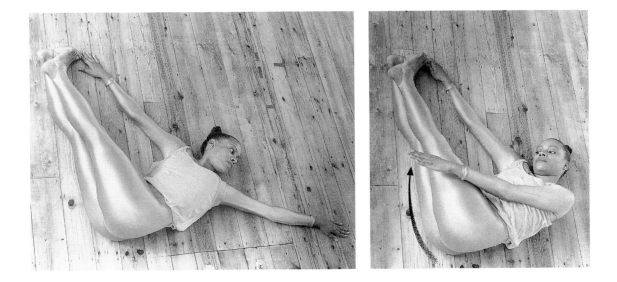

Figure 37: Arm circling on the floor

3. Expand the size of your circles so that your fingers trace an expanding spiral on the floor (Figure 37b).
4. Relax, rest, slowly roll over to the other side and repeat.

Active stretching for more flexibility

Active stretching requires large, fast, throwing movements such as swings and kicks with enough momentum to encourage even further mobility in the joints. Active stretching is for bodies that are fairly supple and sufficiently articulated to withstand this, much stronger, force. The benefits of active stretching are of course a considerable expansion of the movement range. We shall begin with the legs and then proceed to arm movements.

Kicks on the floor

Floor kicks are the most effective way of increasing articulation in the knee and hip joints, as you can kick as high as you please without the hassles of having to balance your body in the upright position or having to carry the weight of your legs against gravity. It is well worth kicking as high as you can because you will be rewarded: once a leg passes the vertical (90 degree) angle, the action becomes easy to do as the weight of your own leg (pulled by gravity) takes the movement further down towards your head all by itself. An added bonus is that these moves also work the stomach and waist muscles.

Figure 38: Floor kicks and gravity: a) against the force of gravity; b) 90-degree point of balance; c) with the force of gravity

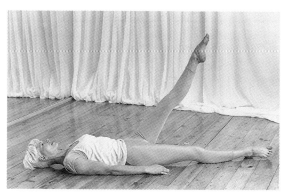

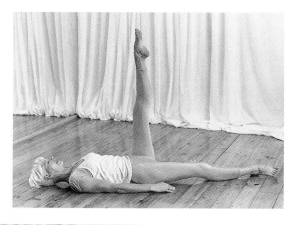

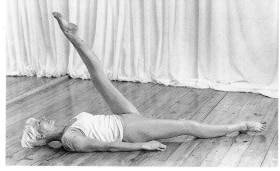

The following sequences of kicks all consist of two moves. Each returns to the same starting position. The first move is a high knee lift, which we call a bent kick, or half kick, followed by 'closing' (bringing the foot back to its original position). The second is a full kick with the knee held straight, followed by closing. A succession of these alternative kicks feels a bit like 'scooping up' something from the floor with your foot. Always breathe in as your leg goes up, out as it comes down.

Forward kicks (Beginners)

1. Lie down on your back, both legs on the floor, bent a little at the knee.
2. Now pull your right knee towards your chest as far as possible. You may, at first, use your hands to help you pull the knee in.
3. Put your right foot back on the floor.
4. Then take a straight kick (with the right leg) upwards, towards the ceiling.
5. Bring it back to the floor.
   Repeat these two alternating moves with the same leg eight to sixteen times. Don't forget to breathe.
6. Rest and repeat with your other leg.

Note: Start the kicks fairly low and, with momentum rather than effort, increase their height until they become larger and larger. Try to attain the height past the vertical and enjoy your leg becoming lighter at its furthest range.

Side kicks (Beginners)

1. Starting position:
   Lie on your right side, bending your right arm so that your head rests on your hand and your armpit faces the floor. Try to place your armpit directly on the floor. If you find it difficult to balance in this straight side-lying position (Figure 39b), then bend your right knee for more stability as shown in Figure 39c. Try to keep your pelvis lying on its side, don't allow your left hip to fall backwards as in Figure 39a.

2. Lift your *left* knee high up towards your left shoulder.
3. Bring your foot back down.
4. Kick your leg straight up towards the ceiling.
5. Bring it back down.

Repeat these kicks eight to sixteen times, one bent, one straight, alternating. You may again increase the height of each kick as you go along until, one day, your leg will touch your head!

Figure 39: Side-lying: a) incorrect; b) balanced; c) with leg support

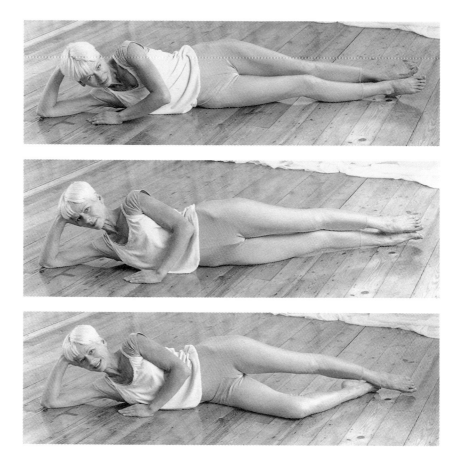

Upper body pivot (Beginners)

1. Still lying on the floor, on your back, pull up your feet and spread your arms out.
2. Using your feet as anchors and the back of your head to move, slide your upper body in a half-circle against the floor so that your upper body moves towards your right hip, while keeping its axis fixed somewhere in your waist area. Try to make a full pivot to the right.
3. Rest and repeat to the left.

Note: Don't lift your head up, keep it on the floor throughout and use it to help you get around. Pivots loosen your bones and tone all the muscles in your back and sides without the painful pressure of gravity.

Lower body pivot

1. Still lying on your back as before, use your shoulders and hips as anchors this time.
2. Take small sideways steps with your feet towards your right side.
3. Keep going until you have completed at least one full circle, or pivot.
4. Repeat to the other side.

Pelvic pivot

1. Still comfortably lying on your back, this time bring your legs up to form a right angle with your waist. Open them wide.
2. Now rotate your pelvis flat on the floor from side to side. Your feet are tracing the two sides of a circle on the ceiling.
3. Gain some momentum in the movement.

Note: Your arms should be outwards on the floor, at shoulder height. All effort to hold your legs should come from your stomach and waist muscles, so relax your neck and shoulders. You might hear a little cracking noise in your spinal vertebrae. That's good. The whole idea is to loosen up any stiff joints in your spine.

Benefits of floor work

A daily stretch, a few kicks and a roll-about on the floor is just as vital for your body as emptying the bowels daily, so don't become physically constipated. From a physical point of view, your body shape will, once again, show the contours of your skeleton, covered in healthy, bouncy muscle. Emotionally, you might like to get rid of some anger and aggression. This can be achieved with the more ferocious kicking movements rather than by screaming at your spouse or kids. But it is now time we got you up from the floor. Wait! How are you going to get up?

Getting up from the floor

On the floor, your circulation and balance are more at ease than when you are standing up. So it is important to submit your body to different levels gradually and smoothly, or you may get dizzy or hurt your back just from getting up too quickly or in the wrong way. Get up slowly, building up the accumulation of weight in your skeleton gradually, from the ground upwards, climbing up each level. Your head always comes last.

1. Roll over, onto your front.
2. Get into crawling position.
3. Sit on your heels.
4. Kneel.
5. Finally step up to standing.

Now your body wants to grow upwards towards its sources of energy, the sun and sky, somewhere beyond the ceiling and the clouds.

1. Stand high up on the balls of your feet (on your toes) and reach up with your fingertips as high as you can. Focus your eyes upwards, like a bud seeking the first rays of spring sunlight.
2. Take a deep breath and lower your heels, lower your arms, relax your shoulders, hands and fingers, but maintain a balanced spine and lifted focus. The energy found in articulation from stretching is now flowing freely in your strong, balanced body.

The Japanese tea ceremony (Advanced)

A more advanced way of getting up from the floor is a move copied from the traditional movements of a Japanese tea ceremony (see Figure 40, pages 98–9). It loosens your knees, strengthens your thigh muscles and improves balance all at once. It will teach you to squat naturally when picking things up. You may not find it so easy to do at first without falling over. If your legs are too weak or too stiff, hold on to something.

Note: Make sure you keep your spine straight and vertical throughout the sequence. If the transition between picture c) and d) proves most difficult at first, practise just this one transitionary movement several times over. It might not work today, but with repeated practice you will soon use this move in your daily life, whenever you have to pick up dirty socks from the floor, or when you have dropped your car keys. Now that you are standing up, let us carry on with some stronger articulation moves.

Articulation – standing

Articulation while standing requires a better sense of balance. If you are a little wobbly at first, have a wall nearby to hold on to just in case. The following swings and kicks will give you a much stronger stance and the stability needed in your trunk to carry larger movements. Be careful: if you have not been swimming or played any outdoor ball games recently you may be a little stiff, so take it slowly to begin with.

Shoulder articulation

This move is not recommended for very stiff people, although just reading it will give a good sense of what it means to try to attain maximum movement range in a joint. The movement begins small and slow, then increases in size and speed until no effort is involved as *momentum* takes over and becomes a powerful stretching force. While this is happening, the joint itself and your whole arm remain relaxed and benefit from an injection of movement energy all the way out as far as the tips of your fingers.

1. Stand with your right foot in front and your left behind in a comfortable stride, keeping your hips square (facing the front). Keep your arms loose and your fingers long. Don't make fists!
2. Swing your left arm in half circles forward and backwards to get it going loosely. Use momentum rather than force. When you feel the extremity of the movement at the top and at the rear, carry on making full *backward* arm circles without moving any other part of your body. Your hand and fingers should lead the action, not your shoulder.

Figure 40: Japanese tea ceremony: a) stand; b) demi plié; *c) toe squat; d) kneel; e) sit on heels; f) kneel; g) point and then sit on feet. Make the return journey to standing in reverse order, starting at g) and finishing at a).*

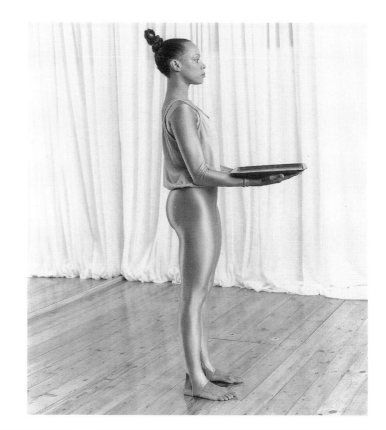

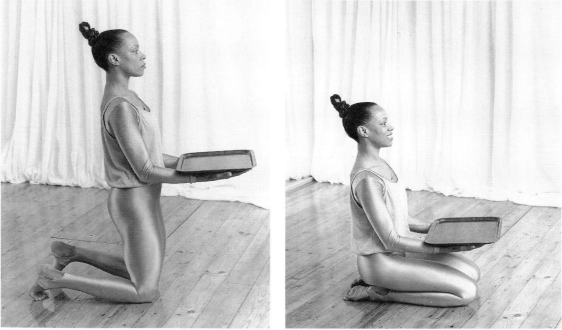

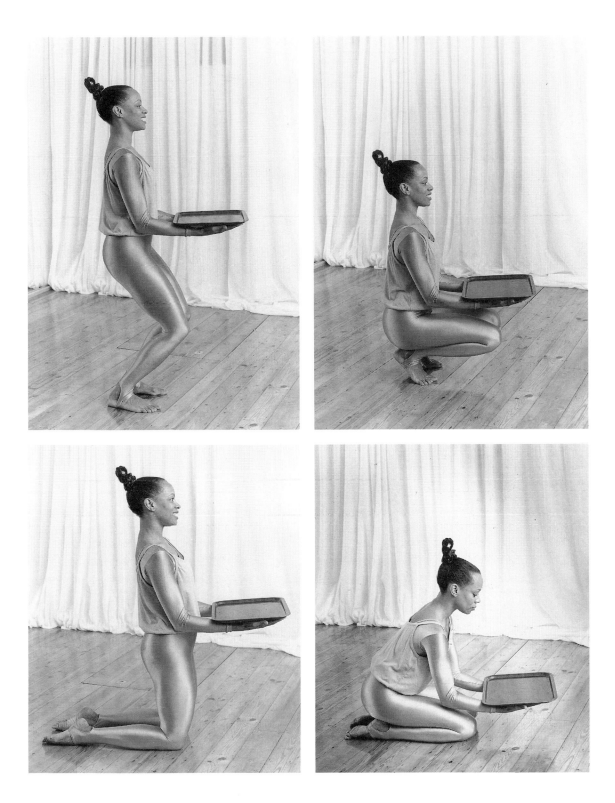

3. Increase the speed of your circular movement until it goes so fast that you feel a tingling sensation in your fingers.
4. When you can absolutely go no faster, hold your arm high above your head for a short moment and shake it gently to let all the blood flow back down to your shoulder.

Change the position of your feet and repeat with your left arm.

Cracking joints, a sign of life

If you feel or hear the odd cracking noise in your shoulder joint, don't worry (provided it doesn't hurt), it is just a sign that things are moving again. Welcome the little noises your body gives you and respond to them with your breathing. These noises are telling you that movement in that region was long overdue. Once you move through the noise a few times, it will stop. Then you will know that the movement range is once more clear and made fully operational. If these cracking noises in your joints persist take a teaspoonful of cod liver oil three times in a week (on alternate days) to 'oil' the hinges of your body. It really does the trick. If you don't like the taste, orange-flavoured cod liver oil can be bought, or get the capsules – but bear in mind that your stomach has to digest the capsules' edible outer plastic-like cover, which you don't really need.

Throwing off upper back and shoulder tension

1. Stand with your feet slightly apart, arms loose by your sides.
2. Look down to your left foot and let your head hang loose in that direction.
3. Now take your right hand and pretend it is a foreign object, a ball or something, and *throw* it over your left shoulder.

Repeat four or six times until the muscles that link your right shoulder to your neck are feeling longer and looser.

Note: It is important to 'throw' your arm and not 'move' it, to allow the force of momentum to work rather than muscle tension, which would only make you stiffer. The reason you are holding your head down towards your opposite foot is to *lengthen* the muscles we are trying to relax. At a more advanced stage this move may be performed with wrist weights to increase its power.

Hanging your spine horizontally (Intermediate)

1. Face a kitchen worktop or other hip-height piece of furniture, standing at least an arm's length away from it.
2. Put your hands on the support and lean down all the way so that your arms are straight and your back is hanging between your tail and your fingers, like a loose net.
   Note: You should feel a pull under your armpits and a feeling of relief in your lower back. Your hamstrings may also be stretching.
3. Now bend and stretch your knees five to eight times to really get to the extremity of your movement range in this position. Your spine will love it.

Figure 41:
Hanging your spine
horizontally

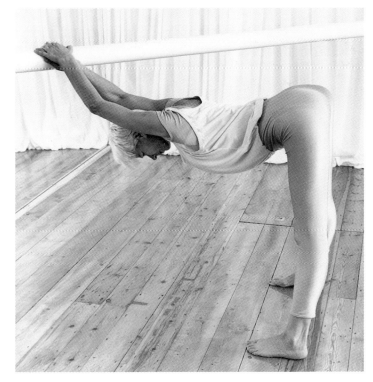

We learned this next move from a very tall and very old Hungaro-Australian chap who, every time he felt a sore back coming on, just got up on his feet and shook his hips like mad with a great sigh of relief. We have therefore named the move after him: the Yuri shake.

Yuri shake

1. Stand up as usual, feet facing front and slightly apart. Keep your arms relaxed.
2. Now shake your hips parallel to the floor as in the old-fashioned dance craze of the fifties, 'the Twist'. The shake should be loose and rapid.

Shaking your leg out

Backache is often caused in part by hip or groin tension. The very deep muscles that line your pelvis cannot be reached with massage or manipulation. The only way to make them 'let go' is simply to shake the tension out.

1. Stand at the top of the stairs, or on a slightly raised surface so that one leg can hang free in mid-air.
2. Shake your free leg by slightly bending your knee and then suddenly stretching your leg downwards. Repeat several times until no more stiff noises can be heard either in your knee, hip or ankle. The shake should feel like you are throwing off a heavy shoe, but in this case the shoe is your foot.

Further articulation moves are given in the next section. They involve quite a lot more power and breath than the moves we have done so far, so if you are feeling tired, close the book and have a rest for now. If you're full of energy, though, read on.

Strength and endurance

Your strength and endurance are determined by your general physical condition and the lifestyle you lead. A heavy body-builder whose body resembles a condom filled with walnuts may look frightfully strong, but his physical condition may not necessarily be enviable. These people are often extremely stiff to the point of being muscle-bound, and can barely move. A professional ballet dancer may not be in top all-round physical shape, either. She might be anorexic and probably has blisters, bunions and corns on her toes. So don't set your sights too high. Remain who *you* are and optimize your condition to give yourself maximum strength and endurance for the things that you want to do. The secret is to have a good balance of movement elements and physical attributes at one's disposal and not to nurture one specific aspect of the body at cost of another.

So far we have covered alignment, balance and articulation. The next thing to brush up is your power, the need for the body to be strong and to exert itself in some way or other. But before getting you to jump around, let's check that your ankles and knees are strong.

You may need:

- a free wall
- a full-length mirror
- a support at hip-height (such as a chest of drawers or chair)
- some mats, cushions and bolsters

It is best, in the beginning, to perform the following moves in front of a full-length mirror to check that you are doing them correctly. Stand near a wall or a piece of furniture so that you can use your arms to help you up and down in case your leg muscles fail.

Ankle power – rises

1. Stand with your feet parallel, shoulder-width apart.
2. Bend your knees to *demi-plié* (your heels are still on the floor).
3. Go up onto the balls of your feet (tip-toes) as high as you can.
4. Go back to *plié*.

Repeat the rise and *plié* eight to sixteen times or more, until your calf muscles feel tired.

Note: Make sure you go up straight by keeping your heels absolutely above your toes, don't allow them to drop out sideways (to sickle). Compare Figure 42a and 42b. Don't take the strain in your shoulders, use your calf and thigh muscles only.

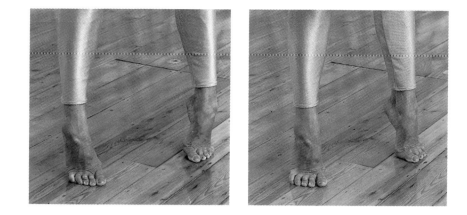

Figure 42: Rise:
a) incorrect;
b) correct

Knee power – squats (Beginners)

The reason a lot of us have difficulty sitting on the floor is that our knees are too stiff and our thigh muscles too weak. The following moves are designed to strengthen these parts of your body. If you regularly wear high-heels, you may not be able to squat fully as your calf muscles will be too short, but it's never too late to regain what nature gave you, so get down to it.

Figure 43: Squats:
a) incorrect;
b) correct

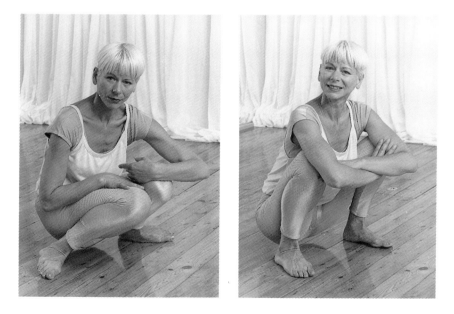

Note: If you cannot manage b), use a band or scarf wound around a steady table leg or some other low attachment, to stop you falling back onto your bum.

Stepping up and down (Intermediate)

You certainly need a couple of soft mats for this, to spare your kneecaps.

1. Stand up, feet slightly apart, toes facing front. Lift your foot arches and relax your knees.
2. Kneel on your right knee.
3. Now both knees.
4. Step up to standing again, leading with your right foot.

Repeat six to eight times or more, until your right thigh muscle begins to get tired. Rest and breathe deeply, then repeat on the other side (this time kneeling down on your left knee first).

Note: The above series of moves are given for bending your legs, squatting, kneeling, and sitting on your heels in various ways. Practise the positions individually as well as moving through the sequence smoothly and effortlessly. This will strengthen your leg and stomach muscles and very soon you will once again, like when you were only two or three years old, feel free, at ease and comfortable on the floor.

Caution: Take special care of the following points:

- Observe the correct vertical placement of your pelvis and spine throughout when you are moving from one position to the next.
- Take strength from your leg muscles, not your shoulders.
- Relax your thorax and breathe deeply to the rhythm of your movements.
- Smile.

Like a proficient ballet dancer, always pretend (on the outside at least) that the movement is easy to do, even if it takes it out of you. Don't let on you are struggling and your struggle will cease as your body achieves accurate muscle control and pure strength.

Now that you have gained some strength in your legs, we may loosen and strengthen your hip joint. This involves much more rigorous action and will also use more lung power, thereby boosting your heart and circulatory system.

Kick your heart out

One of the most widely used moves in dance and movement classes is the kick. A rapid succession of kicks, increasing in height and momentum, has many physiological benefits. First, kicking is the most effective way of increasing articulation in the hip joints while at the same time improving your strength and endurance. Forward kicks specifically work the stomach and thighs, while sideways and backward kicks take care of 'spare tyres' and too much flesh on the hips and bums. So if you really want to lose all that superfluous fat, then get kicking!

Kicks while standing (Intermediate)

The action of kicking requires each leg to function in a different way. One leg becomes the supporting leg while the other is the 'working' leg. It is important in these moves to keep your body weight balanced on the supporting leg while leaving your other leg free to move. The trick in kicks is only to move the leg in action. Doing so demands hard work from many muscles in your whole body. Don't think of a kick as mere leg-work, your whole body is involved. Observe carefully the starting position in Figure 44. While the main move consists of a high kick, the starting position works in the opposite direction and is meant to *lengthen* your calf muscle and Achilles tendon (shown in Figure 44a). This pull is achieved by pressing the heel of your foot firmly into the ground every time it comes down from a kick. From here, your leg is, like a fully drawn catapult, ready to propel a powerful but loose, high kick. When repeated eight or more times, kicks become easier as timing and momentum help the muscles work.

Forward kicks

1. Stand in a lunge, with your right leg bent and your left leg straight behind you, its heel pressed firmly into the floor.
2. Kick your left knee, then your whole leg, returning after each kick to the static position with your left heel firmly pressed into the ground.

Note: Always relax your shoulders. Your supporting leg should be bent while you are standing still and straight as you kick. Make sure the toes of your supporting foot are spread wide, strong and firm, and that your arches are well lifted.

Figure 44: Starting position

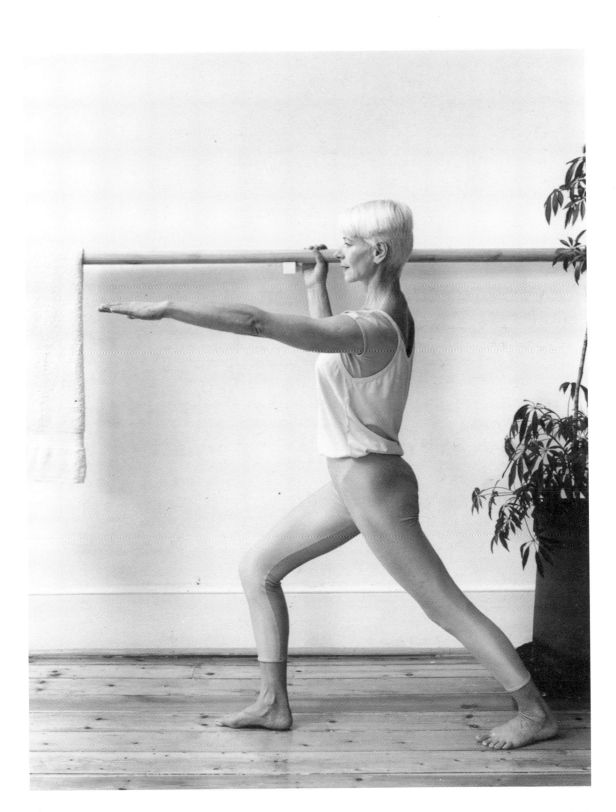

Side kicks (Intermediate)

1. Face the wall and hold on to it with both hands.
2. Alternately kick your knee and then leg out to the side, eight to sixteen times each.

Cloche

Cloche is French for 'bell'. In this movement you pretend that the working leg is a swinging bell. The acquired momentum works with great power on your hip joint while strengthening and stabilizing your spine.

1. Stand by the wall with your weight on your right foot, your left foot on its ball, behind you on the floor. Hold on to the wall with your right hand.
2. Now swing your left leg forwards and backwards, higher and higher until it feels like your foot will fly off on its own.

Note: Make sure you don't move the supporting leg, and relax your shoulders.

Cross kicks (Intermediate)

1. Stand in a wide stride with your arms at shoulder height, a few inches further than shoulder width apart.
2. Kick your right knee across your body to touch your left elbow.
3. Return to the starting position.
4. Now kick your right leg straight across your body to touch your left hand.
5. Return to the starting position again.

Repeat four to eight times, breathe and rest as usual, then cross kick with your left leg.

Wrist and ankle weights (Advanced)

The power of all the preceding articulation moves may be further increased by wearing wrist and/or ankle weights. But be careful, you should always master a move well without weights before trying it with the weights on. So don't be impatient about this. Remember, the whole idea is to let your body guide you in your actions, not to let your own ambitions force your body into impossible situations which might do it more harm than good.

Small jumps (Advanced)

Caution: If your joints hurt or if your neck is not well placed, then do not jump until you have improved your posture. If you feel tall and fit, you may enjoy escaping gravity by jumping. Repeat each of the following combinations between 8 and 32 times, separately or in various sequences, to improve your balance, stamina and brain power.

- Jumping on both feet (bouncing)
- Jumping on one foot (hopping)
- Jumping from one foot to the other (running)
- Standing on both feet, then jumping on one foot (leaping)
- Standing on one foot, then jumping on both feet (assembling)

Lung and heart power

There are many other pleasant ways of reaching full physical power. Although our 'usual' environment doesn't seem very natural or suitable for strong, physical behaviour, it is still possible to train your body during its normal daily to-ings and fro-ings. For example, if you find that you need more lung power, then you should run or jump, or play-fight with your spouse, your children or your dog more often. Or just find a friend to play with. Did you know that laughing is one of the most 'aerobic' types of activities? Laugh yourself into a frenzy, until your tummy aches and you can hardly breathe: it will increase your strength and endurance.

Run for the bus, go by bike instead of by car, or run to your destination when you are in a hurry. Walk or run up the steps next time you use the Underground, rather than taking the lift. Walk to the shops, climb hills, seek fresh air and enjoy a bit of scenery, the cool breeze and some sky at least every day. There are plenty of opportunities to boost your lungs and heart naturally on a daily basis, even in an urban environment. Don't wait until you feel low to remind yourself that your body needs the occasional full-out exertion to stay at the peak of its power. Don't force yourself, but test yourself. You'll be amazed at the strength and stamina you will gain over a short period of time.

Co-ordination and efficiency

Co-ordination entails anything from learning intricate ballroom dancing steps to threading a needle or carrying the breakfast tray from the fourth floor without falling down the stairs. Are you well co-ordinated or are you a somewhat clumsy person? Have you got two left feet? Whatever your state of physical co-ordination, it can always improve. This will save you a lot of time and many accidents. Co-ordination is a matter of your body working out beforehand what it is going to do. Plan your moves with eye movements and thought before you attempt them: 'What am I going to do and how am I going to do it?' In order for an action to be correctly timed and provided with the correct amount of energy, your body has to know in advance the *end goal* of the action. A benefit of good co-ordination and physical awareness is that your body language may be better expressed and understood.

Ambidexterity

The fact that most of us are either right- or left-handed has many detrimental effects on the body. A right-handed person usually leans over a work surface towards the right side. As the right arm is dominant over the left, this also establishes an imbalanced posture. The left leg becomes the 'supporting leg', shifting the balance as a matter of habit over to the left side of the body. This, in turn, causes a slight but permanent deviation in the spine, shoulders and neck, and so the chain of imbalance continues with age, when one eye and one ear get weaker than the others. A very good way of training one's co-ordination is to shift actions from the right hand (if you are right-handed) to the left hand and vice versa. It is a little awkward at first, but forces you to look and feel what your body is actually doing.

Perform the actions listed below with your weaker hand. They will take a little longer, but with a few goes you will soon master them, and in the long run, having two articulate hands instead of just one will help you a lot and save you time. Just give yourself some time to learn and be patient, it will pay off with large dividends.

- Brushing your teeth
- Cutting your nails
- Peeling potatoes
- Writing a post card to a friend
- Threading a needle
- Writing in mirror-image with your good hand, then with the weaker – which is easier?

Upside-down co-ordination

1. Stand a mirror in front of you on the table.
2. Now sit down to write a letter or draw a picture, but look at the motion as it appears in the mirror (that is, upside-down).
3. When you get very good at this, try doing it with your weaker hand.

As for your legs, there is no better way to increase co-ordination than to take up dance lessons. So if you are the kind of person who habitually walks like a drunken elephant, knocking into things all the time and frequently losing your balance, then take an amateur dance course. There are many styles to choose from, suitable for any age group. You won't feel inhibited, as all participants join for the same reasons: to improve their bodies and to have fun. Just pick one to suit your taste, from folk dancing to ballroom, tap, jazz, jive, rock & roll, ballet, belly dancing, etc. Even some forms of martial arts such as T'ai Chi, kendo, karate and capeiorea are all excellent for co-ordination practice.

To test your arm co-ordination skills, try the following arm swings.

Counter-circles

1. Stand up with your arms loose by your sides.
2. Start swinging your arms forward and backwards as you do when walking.
3. Make the swings larger and larger until they become circles. Your arms should be circling in opposite directions: your right arm going up and backwards while your left is coming down and forward. Also try it the other way round. Good luck!

Figure 45:
Counter-circles

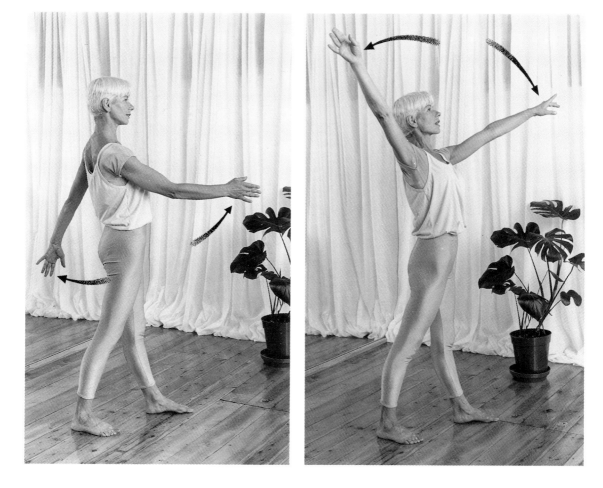

Recovery

Counter moves

With the best will in the world it still happens that the body gets abused, is made to sit, stand, hang or lean in an unfavourable position for too long. This happens mostly when you are engaged in mental activity which requires long periods of concentration. The brain seems to take over, forgetting that the body is in real discomfort, until you stand up and feel the pain. A useful thing to know is that wherever the pain came from, if you have noted the position the body was in that caused this pain, then you are also able to get the body out of it again, often instantly. The simple answer is to make a *counter move* with the body.

If, for example, you have been leaning over a computer for two hours, the remedial position would be a backward bend. Increased backward mobility in the spine is essential for balance and should be cultivated in two stages.

Bending back

As most actions in daily life occur in front of your body, curving or hanging backwards is the only movement that will straighten your spine after an overdose of sitting, looking, or concentrating on the everyday things you do with your hands and head. Like a flower that is turned to face the light, allow your body to grow up and back, to balance and be tall. As a rule, if you don't want to grow shorter and begin to bend downwards, prematurely towards the grave, for each forward bend your body makes, a backward bend should follow to cancel out the growing habitual imbalance of your body.

First your spine must be made loose and mobile again. This can be done effortlessly by lying on your back, relaxing over a curved surface or a partner's legs as illustrated in Figure 46. You may use a large bolster or cushion instead of a partner, or even the top of a well-carpeted staircase to curve your spine backwards.

It is important at this stage not to attempt to bend backwards in the upright position as the muscles required to hold you up are not trained yet. In addition, the muscles at your solar plexus (diaphragm) are too short to allow backward-bending and need to be passively and gently stretched before any effort is demanded from them. They would cramp, hurt and discourage you from repeating the action.

Passive backward-bending

1. Lie down over your chosen support and bring your arms up high above your head, stretching your fingers out fully.
2. Lie back and breathe deeply or, even better, sing to keep your throat open in this unfamiliar position. If you feel dizzy and begin to see stars, it means that your upper back and neck are stuck and therefore need this type of movement. But take it gently. Support your head with a hand or cushion. Lengthen and relax the back of your neck and breathe in deeply. Keep your chin down or you might cut off the oxygen supply to your brain and become dizzy again. Sleeping with a small beauty pillow (see page 32) will also improve the condition.

Figure 46: Passive backward-bending; recovery positions: a) incorrect; b) correct

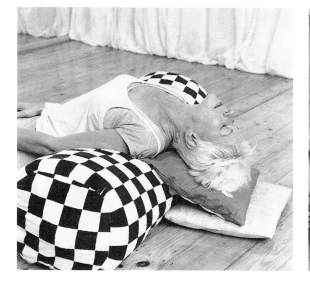 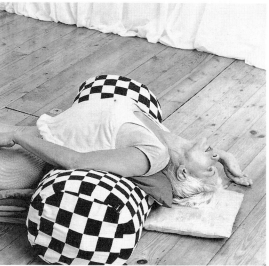

Recovering from a backward bend

When you decide to come out of the position, don't get up quickly. Gently roll over onto your side, crawl on all fours, sit on your heels, and stand up as shown on page 95, head last.

Bending back while standing (Intermediate)

Figure 47: Bending back with support

Now that your skeleton has been made mobile through passive, supported bending, you may attempt bending back while upright. An easy way to begin is to hold on to something while letting your body hang from your arms.

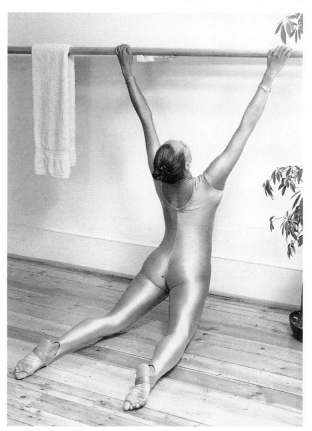

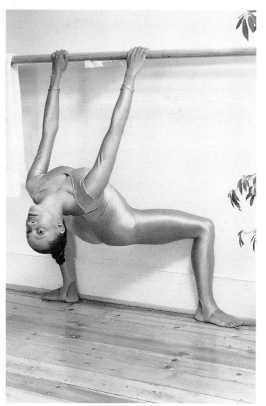

In a slightly more demanding backward bend your hands may be used for support at the back of your head, your waist and/or the back of your legs.

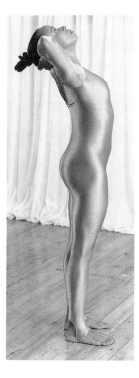

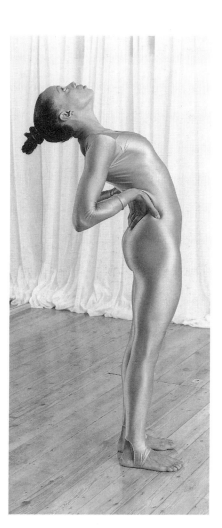

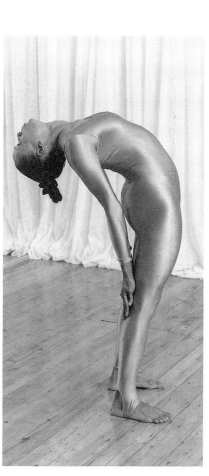

Figure 48: Bending back using your hands for support: a) head; b) waist; c) legs

Hanging back by your arms

At a more advanced stage, hanging from a trapeze or door frame is even more enjoyable. Lift your head and look up. How far up and back can you see? Don't forget to keep your neck long, to breathe and/or sing.

Figure 49: Hanging back by your arms

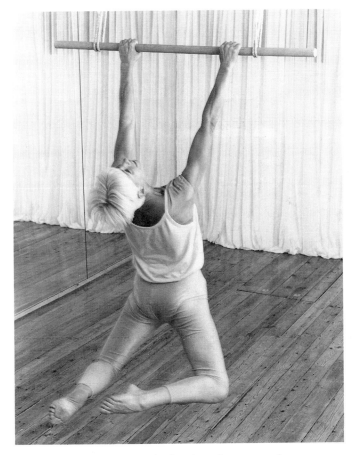

To loosen your spine further, here are three progressive moves to practise. Don't attempt the impossible, though. Try the Fish first, then the Crab, and then, if you really want more, attempt to stretch your legs while in the Crab position to achieve the perfect Bridge.

Fish

Your elbows are supporting your waist, your neck is relaxed.

Figure 50: Fish

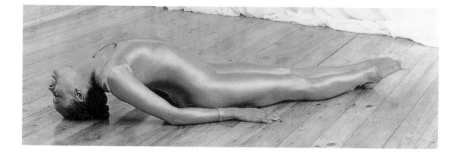

Crab (Intermediate)

Position your hands as shown in Figure 51, with your fingers *pointing in towards your body* before you start.

Figure 51: Crab

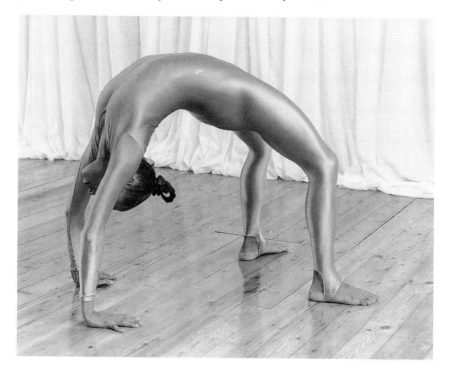

Bridge (Advanced)

Figure 52: Bridge

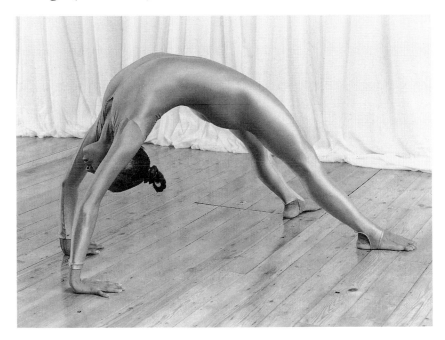

Take the trouble to recondition your upper back daily, especially if you have been sitting a lot. Don't spend more time on chairs than necessary. Enjoy your floor at home and wherever permissible.

For partners

All the skills learned so far can now be put into practice with other people. A partner session is not unlike 'contact improvisation', a form of modern dance in which the partners' body-weights are merged, shared and thrown about playfully.

Together with a partner of any age, sex or creed you may try testing your sense of your own direction and weight. Focus on your partner's body. Sometimes your mutual weight will be shared, sometimes given or taken, bounced between you like a

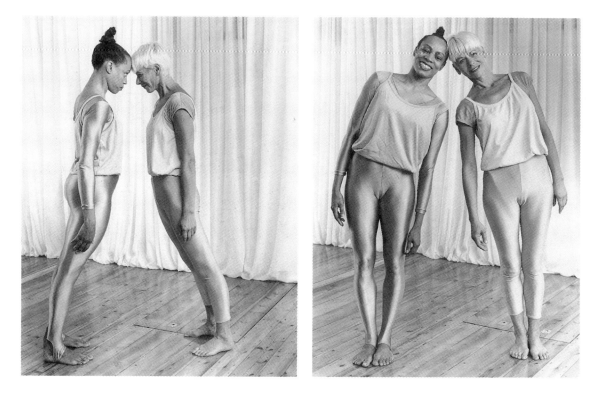

Figure 53:
Leaning turn

ball or lost altogether in feelings of surprise and ecstasy. You will both have a lot of fun.

Turning together (Beginners)

This move always makes people laugh, as it reminds them of their youth. What you didn't know as a child was that it also releases much tension and improves your circulation and balance.

1. Face each other and join hands. Stretch your arms out fully and lean back.
2. Start turning, slowly, then faster and faster.

Note: Lean well back and straighten your elbows. Your feet need hardly move at all. Turn again in the opposite direction so you don't get dizzy.

Leaning turn (Intermediate)

1. Stand facing your partner about a 3 ft/1 m apart. Now lean towards each other from your legs up (not from your bum)

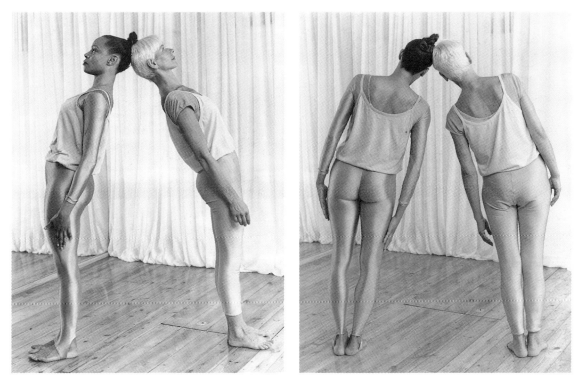

until your foreheads touch. Keep your arms by your sides and your body stiff (Figure 53a).

2. Now each of you should turn on the spot in opposite directions, a quarter turn at a time, as follows:

3. A quarter-turn away from each other (Figure 53b).

4. Another quarter-turn (you are now back to back, still leaning into one another and heads touching) (Figure 53c).

5. Another quarter-turn (you are now side by side, still leaning with your heads together and keeping your bodies straight from head to toe) (Figure 53d).

6. Finally, turn the last quarter to face one another again as in the starting position.

'Spotting' your partner's eyes (1) (Intermediate)

This move will improve your balance, circulation and sense of direction. In addition, it will loosen your upper back and neck. The means of achieving this is to 'spot', or focus on, your partner's eyes.

1. Stand about 10 ft/3 m apart, facing each other. Stand close to a wall so that you can hold on to it if you lose your balance.
2. Look each other in the eyes and begin to turn, but try to *maintain eye contact*.

Note: Observe the direction of your turns. If one partner is turning clockwise, the other has to turn anti-clockwise. Try the move slowly at first while holding on to something.

'Spotting' your partner's eyes (2) (Advanced)

When you can both turn around fully without losing eye contact, you can try doing it closer together, away from the wall. Eventually, when done faster and closer together still, the turn becomes a classic Spanish duet turn. Have fun with it.

Partner massage

In partner massage there is always an active person and a passive person. Yet the person who is being massaged should not just lie there like a dead turkey. His or her breathing (if nothing else) can give the masseur or masseuse valuable hints as to how the session is progressing. Be relaxed, but don't be afraid to communicate your feelings or readjust your position. It helps the masseur or masseuse to know whether what he or she is doing is any good for you. Where is the pain? Should the pressure be harder or softer, faster or slower? A massage is a subtle collaboration between two people. A good massage benefits both partners' bodies. A good masseur or masseuse uses body weight with the force of gravity.

Using body weight rather than force

Never use unnecessary force. For example, if you are massaging someone's back and want to reach the deep muscles, you need to exert quite a large amount of force. But rather than just pushing and pounding with your hands and arms, add pressure by using your body weight instead. Lean into the position and the force of gravity will be transmitted effortlessly. Similarly, when it is necessary to pull on a limb to make it more loose in its socket, lean away so that a pulling force is created naturally by gravity rather than by your own muscle strength.

Using your feet

In addition to the conventional type of massage which is done mostly with the hands, there are other forms of massage that use other parts of the body – the feet, for example – to apply force.

A good way to begin might be to have someone smaller than yourself, even your child, gently walk all over you while you are lying face-down on the floor. Make sure he or she doesn't walk directly on your spine or behind your knee joints. If this is done by a small child it will also give him or her a reassuring feeling that adults, too, can be small, low down, vulnerable and sensitive. You will gain respect for this while the child will become more self-assured. An adult partner can work just as well, but of course should not use his or her full body weight, but rather just one foot, perhaps, or some other part of his or her body.

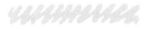

Full body contact

A natural progression from the hand, foot/body part massage is contact work in which the partners share their entire body weight.

Upper back and neck loosener (Beginners)

1. Partner A sits on the floor, legs straight out in front.
2. Partner B lies down with shoulder blades across Partner A's legs and arms raised above the head to create a slight backward curve at the top of the spine. Relax.
3. Partner A gently shakes the legs to give Partner B a jolly good wobble in this relaxed backward position.
4. At this point we usually hear a pleasant 'Aaahhh' sound of relief coming from Partner B as some upper back tension is released. Now Partner B is only too willing to swap places and share this new experience.

Such moves may be performed at any time when you are leisurely relaxing about the house.

Caution: One thing should be borne in mind here. Don't allow the 'passive' partner to bend his or her neck back too sharply as this would defeat the object of the move, which is to make the neck longer and freer. If your partner's neck is too stiff, support

Figure 54: Upper back and neck loosener:

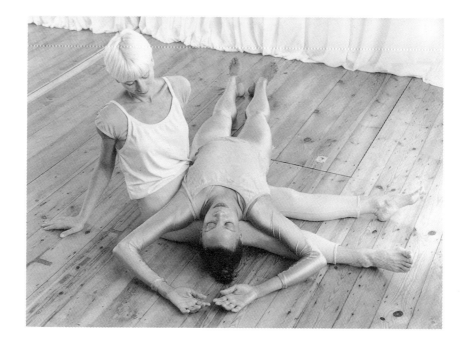

it in the beginning with your hand or a small cushion to keep his or her neck long and straight.

Back-to-back stretch (Intermediate)

1. Sit back-to-back on the floor, with no gap between your two lower spines. Push your bums close together and make sure your spines and the backs of your heads are touching.
2. Partner A bends the knees and leans back over Partner B, who lowers the body down towards the legs.

Note: Don't join hands and both relax. Stay in the position calmly breathing until you both feel you want to get out of it.

3. Return to sitting up.
4. Repeat the action in reverse to stretch Partner A's hamstrings and curve Partner B's spine backwards.

Note: Make sure that a) both your bodies are fully relaxed at the end of the movement and b) that your bums, backs and heads are in full contact and are supported by your partner when you bend back.

Figure 55: Back-to-back stretch

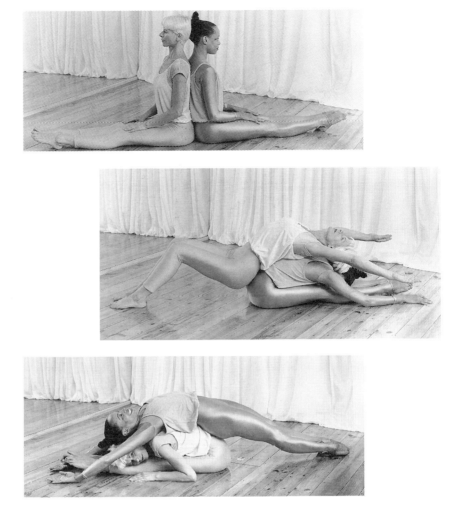

Sandwich

The sandwich is literally child's play for two fairly equal-sized bodies.

1. Partner A lies face-down on the floor and is told: 'You are the bread.'
2. Partner B lies face-up on top of Partner A and is told: 'You are the butter.'

For groups

Multi-decker people-burger

Now, if there are any more willing participants, the sandwich may be garnished with 'cheese', 'tomatoes', 'mayonnaise', etc. to make a veritable multi-decker people-burger. A mixture of adult and children's bodies in varying sizes can be fun – usually ending up with a whole pile of laughing people rolling apart like a stack of logs. This game is definitely recommended as a family pastime or as a party trick.

Figure 56: Multi-decker people-burger

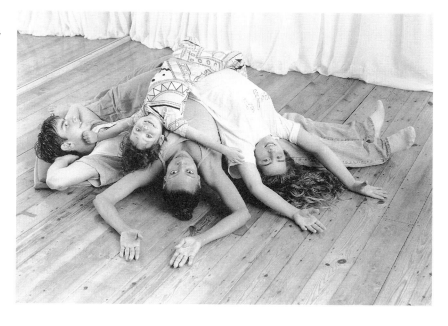

Lapsit for two (Intermediate)

While you are having fun with your friends, why not pair up and try the lapsit for two? We learned this move from a 1960s San Franciscan movement called 'New Games'. Their motto is 'Play hard, play fair, nobody hurt'. Choose a partner roughly your own size and:

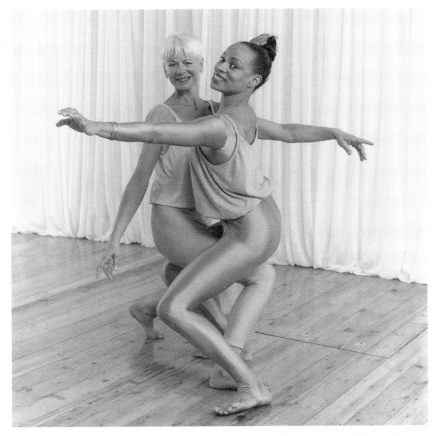

1. Stand facing each other touching in a shoulder-width stride so that your feet are positioned as shown in Figure 57.
2. Now embrace and slowly bend at the knees to end up sitting on each other's laps. Trust that you can share gravity and still be balanced together. Stop laughing or you might fall. Relax.
3. When you have secured your mutual balance (somehow), let go of each other's hands and lift your arms high up in the air.

Lapsit for many (Beginners)

Read the instructions carefully and no one will fall, yet the group will discover a new sense of bonding and security, ease and comfort. Apparently, the world record in lapsitting was achieved by 1468 people in Palmito del Verde, Mexico. Try it with between *5 and 15 people* of fairly equal size. If there are youngsters in the group, put them inside the circle and promise them a special treat at the end of the game.

1. Stand shoulder to shoulder in a circle.
2. Now everybody make a quarter-turn to the right and place your hands on the waist of the person in front of you.
3. Take a side step with your left foot to tighten the circle.
4. Now gently ease and guide the person in front of you onto your lap while you yourself also lower your weight onto the lap of the person behind you.

That's all! Are you sitting comfortably?

5. Everyone shakes hands with the kids in the middle. If there are no children playing, reach into the circle and all shake hands together.
6. Stand up (careful, now!), break the circle, have a giggle and a chat, then try it again facing left.

Figure 58: Lapsit for many

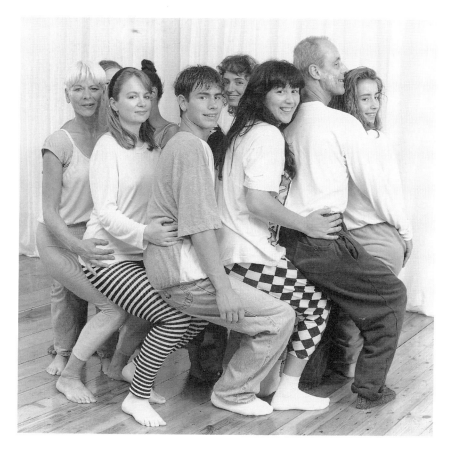

There is not enough room in this book to mention the number of games you can play. The more you play, the more you free your body from its tensions and inhibitions. By inventing many more games for two or more bodies, be they children, partners, parents or friends, you will discover many new wonderful sensations.

Kando in your life

It is not only possible but also easy to change. The Kando technique helps you learn to reconstruct, feel and understand how your body works and what it wants to do. You have seen how ingrained habits can easily be programmed out and replaced with more efficient and economic moves. Studying human movement turns out to be far less complex and convoluted than it might have seemed. Experienced observers can always tell by a subject's movements what that person is feeling. 'The body doesn't lie,' said Martha Graham, the best-known modern dance choreographer of the twentieth century. Our verbal language can often be negated or contradicted by our physical behaviour.

Many politicians and media people are now trained by public relations companies on how to control their body language. Sharpening up your powers of observation helps you recognize the true meaning of physical expression. The movement dynamics or qualities found in a person's physical behaviour usually match his or her personality and moods. Find out what your movement style is, and try to train it to meet the feelings of each moment with competence, grace, fluency and sincerity.

Put your brain in your toes

The brain is just another organ and has its functions like any other: it processes your thoughts, actions and emotions. Just as if you eat bad food or breathe bad air you are going to suffer, your brain will suffer if you think bad thoughts or expose yourself to situations that cause negative feelings. Similarly, if you don't use your brain it will atrophy (become useless, dormant).

Up until quite recently scientists regarded the brain as a ruling organ, the regulator, information distributor – in short the boss over all other organs. We now know that the substance the brain is made of is also found in the spine, the solar plexus (diaphragm) and in every bone in your body near the points of articulation. What then, gives the brain the monopoly on intelligence? And indeed, quantum physics shows that every molecule in the body has intelligence. For years now we have been asking our clients to 'put their brains in their toes' to help them place their feet better. Perhaps the idea was not so crazy after all. If the area behind the neck is permanently bent and blocked, it creates a veritable traffic jam along the brain/body motorway. Poor carriage of the head, as happens when posture is poor, causes the neck to fold and 'strangulate' the brain stem – where nerves for movement, touch, taste, smell and feeling are located.

Now that you have decongested the area at the back of your neck and located your brain stem, you may discover a link between your brain and the rest of your body, and may decide that comfort, health, beauty and efficiency are largely determined by the number of moves you have at your disposal for acting, living and expressing yourself.

The laws of movement are beyond verbal description and analysis. That is why the bulk of this book gives you *moves* and illustrations rather than complicated-and-very-nearly-correct-but-in-the-end-quite-meaningless-and-ineffective-analyses. While it is possible nowadays to obtain a scientific degree at the highest level in dance and physical education, and there may be 20 different words for one body part or a single action, *movement is simple and subtle*, limited only by the body's anatomy and condition. Each person has only one head, a trunk and four limbs to cope with. A raised hand may hold a gun or a bunch of flowers, but the act of lifting the arm is fundamentally the same.

The Kando technique is best learned by doing. Play with your family, friends, pets and don't forget to play with your toes and your fingers. Keep yourself mobile and agile without getting unnecessarily tired. The mysteries of body language will unfold in your natural physical reactions and interactions, guided by your senses. The moves and ideas given in this book are of course only a beginning. We hope they will form a basic vocabulary of possibilities to equip you to explore and invent many more, new ways of carrying yourself in the world. It is now up to you, having now reached the end of the book, to continue the never-ending journey towards a bit more elegance, tolerance, open-mindedness and, last but not least, greater comfort and ease to help you achieve the most important goals in your life.

Among the many letters we receive, one in particular describes what the technique is really about. It came from a friend called Gerda in Amsterdam (this excerpt has been translated from the Dutch).

The pleasure your body feels goes to your mind: it is something we all have in us but do not always realize. If you pay careful attention to how your body reacts, you get to know which moves are good for you. It is good to exert yourself physically, to perhaps once a day make your heart beat faster, even if it is only by walking up some stairs. It is a miracle what you can do with your body, how willing it is and how happy it is that you give it some attention by, for example, making it feel muscles that were never used come back to life again. Your body picks up very quickly and soon brings what it learns into its own daily movement patterns, without having to think about it. And the biggest surprise is that, on top of all this, the body transmits all its gratitude, happiness and enthusiasm to the mind, which in turn becomes clearer, opens itself more fully, as it were, and through all this extra enthusiasm of body and mind – which happens all by itself, without effort – you become completely renewed and especially happy with yourself.

Like Gerda and so many others who have become more familiar with the technique, you will discover that helping yourself to develop your body and your brain is fun, and this will become your favourite pastime. Achieving results in one area is gratifying and encourages you to continue. Improvement now prevents premature ageing and complications or trouble later on in life. Treat your vehicle for life, your body, with respect and learn to improve its performance, then it will never age disgracefully. We cannot make you immortal. But *you* can turn the usual chain of events literally on its head. You too can be like our own grandmother, who was still working and swimming at 98 years of age. You can stay active and creative and enjoy your friends' and children's respect way past maturity in this fascinating physical world we all share for a while.

Daily, weekly and monthly progress chart

Y ou might like to photocopy this chart to mark the moves you are working on, starting a new chart from time to time so you can measure your progress. Most moves are suitable for any level of fitness. The more demanding ones are marked *(int.)* for intermediate and *(adv.)* for advanced. Page numbers are given for easy reference.

Choose two new moves to learn every day from the 'daily' column. Once a week add a move from the 'weekly' column, and once a month check that you can still do a choice of those marked in the 'monthly' column.

For tuition in the Kando technique, teacher training or a catalogue of 'body-friendly' equipment, please send a s.a.e. to one of our head offices:

UK/EUROPE

Kando Studios
88 Victoria Road
London NW6 6QA
Tel. 071–625 6577

USA

Kando Studios
4 Elmbrook Circle
Bedford, MA
01730
Tel. (617) 275-3690

Move	Daily	Weekly	Monthly	Page
Hips, bums, tums and thighs				
Couches built into your body	●			38
TV-watching positions	●			39
Baby pose	●			54
Breakfast move: Licking the plate (*int.*)		●		55
For fat legs and ankles (water retention)	●			55
Are you chairbound?			●	57
Feeling the sitting bones	●			59
Sitting on your own built-in seat	●			59
Bum racing			●	60
Wobble, wobble all fall down		●		60
Spinning top (*int.*)		●		60
Back, neck, shoulders and face				
Baby pose with turn-out		●		64
Baby pose with one leg outstretched	●			65
Baby pose with one leg bent to the side			●	65
Correct neck alignment (*adv.*)	●			66
Lengthening the torso		●		66
Horizontal twist	●			67
Ironing out your spine (*int.*)	●			67
Shoulder stand (*adv.*)			●	68
Safe sun-focusing		●		70
Pirouette with the sun (*int.*)			●	70
Realignment				
Quarter rolls with balance and flop		●		71
Quarter rolls with kicks (*int.*)		●		72
Quarter rolls with body curve (*adv.*)			●	73
Continuous rolling	●			73
Stance and balance				
Foot alignment	●			75
Bouncing	●			76
Building a balanced posture	●			76
Shoulder placement	●			77
Neck and head placement	●			78

Move	Daily	Weekly	Monthly	Page
Standing spinal twists		●		78
Turning on the spot		●		79
Dervish turn (*int.*)			●	80
Articulation — lying down				
Toe-pulling	●			81
Moving your ankles	●			82
Moving your knees	●			82
Loosening your knees		●		82
Stretching your hamstrings	●			83
Turn-out		●		84
One-legged turn-in	●			87
Turn-out and turn-in		●		87
Sitting on your heels	●			88
Folding your legs under (*adv.*)			●	89
Circling your leg		●		90
Arm circling on the floor		●		90
Forward kicks		●		93
Side kicks		●		93
Upper body pivot			●	94
Lower body pivot			●	95
Pelvic pivot			●	95
Getting up from the floor	●			95
Japanese tea ceremony (*adv.*)		●		96
Articulation — standing				
Shoulder articulation		●		97
Throwing off upper back and shoulder tension		●		100
Hanging your spine horizontally (*int.*)	●			101
Yuri shake		●		102
Shaking your leg out			●	102
Strength and endurance				
Ankle power — rises	●			103
Knee power — squats	●			104
Stepping up and down (*int.*)		●		105
Forward kicks		●		106
Side kicks (*int.*)		●		108
Cloche		●		108

Move	Daily	Weekly	Monthly	Page
Cross kicks (*int.*)	●			108
Small jumps (*adv.*)		●		109
Co-ordination and efficiency				
Ambidexterity	●			100
Upside-down co-ordination			●	111
Counter-circles			●	112
Recovery				
Passive backward-bending	●			114
Recovering from a backward bend	●			115
Bending back while standing		●		115
Hanging back by your arms		●		117
Fish		●		118
Crab (*int.*)			●	118
Bridge (*adv.*)			●	119
For partners				
Turning together			●	120
Leaning turn (*int.*)		●		120
'Spotting' your partner's eyes (1) (*int.*)		●		121
'Spotting' your partner's eyes (2) (*adv.*)			●	122
Partner massage		●		122
Using body weight rather than force	●			122
Using your feet			●	123
Upper back and neck loosener		●		123
Back-to-back stretch			●	124
Sandwich			●	125
For groups				
Multi-decker people-burger		●		126
Lapsit for two (*int.*)			●	126
Lapsit for many			●	127

Bibliography

Irmgard Bartenieff and Dori Lewis, *Body Movement: Coping with the Environment* (Gordon & Breach Science Publishers, New York, Paris, London, 1980).

Ben E. Benjamin, *Are You Tense? The Benjamin System of Muscular Therapy* (Pantheon Books, New York, 1978).

Itzhak Bentov, *Stalking the Wild Pendulum: On the Mechanics of Consciousness* (Wildwood House, London, 1978).

Norma Canner, *. . . And a Time to Dance* (Plays Inc., Boston, Mass., 1975).

Janice M. Cauwels, *Bulimia, the Binge-Purge Compulsion* (Doubleday & Co., Inc., Garden City, New York, 1983).

Martha Davis and Jane Skupien, *Body Movement and Nonverbal Communication: an Annotated Bibliography, 1971-80* (Indiana University Press, Bloomington, Indiana, 1982).

Ed van der Elsken and Eddy Postuma de Boer, *Dans Theatre* (A. W. Bruna & Zoon, 1960).

Ed van der Elsken, *Eye Love You* (Van Holkema & Warendorf, Bussum, 1977).

Moshe Feldenkrais, *Awareness Through Movement* (Harper & Row, New York, San Francisco, London, 1972).

John H. Flavell, *Cognitive Development* (Prentice Hall, Englewood Cliffs, New Jersey, 1977).

Andrew Fluegelman (ed.), *The New Games Book* (Sidgwick & Jackson, 1978).

Raoul Gelabert, *Anatomy for the Dancer: with exercises to improve technique and prevent injuries* (Dance Magazine Inc., New York, 1964).

Michael Gelb, *An Introduction to the Alexander Technique* (Aurum Press, London, 1981, 1987).

Charles J. Golden, PhD, *Current Topics in Rehabilitation Psychology* (Grüne & Stratton, Orlando, Florida, 1984).

Vivian Grisogono, *Sports Injuries* (John Murray (Publishers) Ltd, 1984–6).

Dr Maria Hári et al., *Scientific Studies on Conductive Pedagogy* (Institute for Conductive Education of the Motor Disabled Conductor's College, Budapest, 1975).

Malcolm Hulke (ed.), *The Encyclopedia of Alternative Medicine and Self-Help* (Schocken Books, New York, 1979).

Michael Hutchison, *Mega Brain* (Ballantine Books, New York, 1987).

Brian Inglis and Ruth West, *The Alternative Health Guide* (Knopf, New York, 1983).

Juliette Kando, 'Co-ordination', *New Dance Magazine*, Feb. 1982.

——, 'The Foot and your Health', *The Dance Teacher*, 38, 2, 3, Feb.–Mar. 1989.

——, *The Natural Face Book* (Thorsons, 1991).

Thomas M. Kando, *Leisure and Popular Culture in Transition* (The C. V. Mosby Company, St. Louis, Toronto, 1980).

——, *Sexual Behaviour and Family Life in Transition* (Elsevier/North Holland Inc., 1978).

Frank H. Krusen, MD, Frederic J. Kottke, MD, PhD and Paul M. Ellwood, Jr, MD, *Handbook of Physical Medicine and Rehabilitation* (W.B. Saunders Co., Philadelphia, London, Toronto, 1971).

Michio Kushi, *The Macrobiotic Way of Natural Healing* (East West Publications, Boston, Mass., 1978).

Lucinda Lidell, Sata Thomas, Carola Beresford Cooke and Anthony Porter, *The Book of Massage* (Simon & Schuster, 1984).

Lucy Lidell, *The Book of Yoga* (Ebury Press, 1983).

Jack Maguire, *Care and Feeding of the Brain: a Guide to your Grey Matter* (Doubleday, New York, 1990).

Desmond Morris, Peter Collett, Peter Marsh and Marie O'Shaughnessy, *Gestures* (Stein & Day, New York, 1979).

Marion North, *Body Movement for Children: an Introduction to Movement Study and Teaching* (Plays, Inc., Boston, Mass. 1971).

——, *Personality Assessment through Movement* (Plays, Inc., Boston, Mass., 1975).

Helen Payne (ed.), *Dance Movement Therapy: Theory and Practice* (Routledge, 1992).

Valerie Preston-Dunlop, *Practical Kinetography Laban* (Dance Horizon, Inc., New York, 1969).

Ruth Purtilo, *Health Professional/Patient Interaction* (W.B. Saunders Co., Philadelphia, London, Toronto, 1984).

Pamela Ramsden, *Top Team Planning: A Study of the Power of Individual Motivation in Management* (Associate Business Programmes Ltd., London, 1973).

M. S. Sanders and E. J. McCormick, *Human Factors in Engineering and Design* (McGraw-Hill International Editions, 1987).

Celia Sparger, *Anatomy and Ballet* (Theatre Arts Books, New York, 1970).

E. Winifred Thacker, MCSP, *Postural Drainage and Respiratory Control* (Lloyd Luke, 1959).

Alan B. Wallace, *Choosing Reality: A Contemplative View of Physics and the Mind* (Shambala Publications Inc., Boston, Mass., 1989).

Bernice K. Watt and Annabel L. Merrill, *Composition of Foods* (US Department of Agriculture, Washington DC, 1975).

Fred Alan Wolf, *The Body Quantum: The New Physics of Body, Mind and Health* (Heinemann, London, 1986).

Index

Achilles tendon 106
active stretching 91
aerobics 109
Alexander 13
alignment, neck 66
ambidexterity 110
ankle power – rises 103
ankles, moving your 82
ante/postnatal depression 14
arches
    cross 76
    long 75
arm circling on the floor 90
articulation
    lying down 81
    shoulder 97
    standing 97

babies 17
baby pose 54
    with one leg bent to the side 65
    with one leg outstretched 65
    with turn-out 64
back
    bending your upper back 114
    how to cure your bad back 64
    hanging back from the arms 117
    horizontal spinal twist 67
    passive backward bending 114
    throwing off tension 100
    upper back and neck loosener 123
backache 21, 102
back, neck, shoulders and face 64
back-to-back stretch 124
balance 74, 120
    building a balanced posture 76
    sense of 19
balancing 19
basic wardrobe 29
beauty pillow 32
bending back 113
    while standing 115
bingeing shop-aholic 48
'body-friendly' equipment 30

body weight 122
bolster
    giant 34
    hard 30
bouncing 76
bowel motion 50
bras 27
breakfast move: licking the plate 55
bridge 119
building a balanced posture 76
built-in seat 59
bum racing 60

canvas strap 32
cellulite 55
chair 25, 43
chairbound 57
charts, progress 134
chewing 52
Children's Arts Corner 14
choreography 44
circling your legs 90
classical dance 12
cloche 108
cod liver oil 100
coils 28
comfort, dressing for 25
contact, full body 123
continuous rolling 73
co-ordination and efficiency 110
correct neck alignment 66
counter-circles 112
counter moves 113
crab 118
cracking joints 100
cross kicks 108

depression 21
Dervish turn 80
desk work 41
drinking 52

E.T.D. 45
efficiency 110

emotional trauma 21
emotional traumatic disorder (E.T.D.) 45
enzymes 52
ergonomic hints
  in the kitchen 39
  in the lounge 38
ergonomics 36

face 70
fashion 27
fat 48
fat legs and ankles (water retention) 55
feeling the sitting bones 59
fish 118
fitness 16
flexibility 90
floor
  getting up from the 95
  kicks 91
  mat 30
  work, benefits of 95
folding your legs under 89
foot alignment 75
force 122
forward kicks 93, 106
foundations 75
freedom of movement 27
fruit 51
full body contact 123
full-length mirror 24
furniture 25
  built in your own body 59

genetically inherited movements 10
getting up from the floor 95
glasses 28
gloves 28
gravity 9, 74
groin tension 84
groups 126

hammock 33
hamstrings 57
  stretching 83
handbags 28
hands 35
hanging back by the arms 117
hanging your spine horizontally 101
hats 28
head placement 78
heart 42
  power 109
high heels 26
hip joint, articulation of the 83
hips, bums, tums and thighs 54, 60
horizontal twist 67

ironing out your spine 67

Japanese Tea Ceremony 96
jewellery 28
joints, cracking 100
jumps, small 109

kicks
  cross 108
  floor 91
  forward 93, 106
  side 93, 106

while standing 106
knee power – squats 104
knees
  loosening 82
  moving 82

lapsit for many 127
lapsit for two 126
laughing 18
leaning turn 120
leg, shaking out 102
legs, circling 90
lengthening the torso 66
lighting 45
long coats 28
loosening your knees 82
lower body pivot 95
lung and heart power 109

M.E. 37, 45
massage
  partner 122
  self 35
  using your feet 123
mats 30
meat 50
migraine 21, 74
mirror
  angled 34
  full-length 24
morning sickness 14
motherhood 14
moving your ankles 82
moving your knees 82
multi-decker people-burger 126
muscles
  on the shin 26
  thigh 104
  unused 49
music and sound 44
myalgic encephalomyelitis (M.E.) 37, 45

neck alignment 66
negative habits 11
nuts 59

office, at the 41
one-legged turn-in 87

partner massage 122
passive articulation 64
passive backward bending 114
passive stretching 16
pelvic pivot 95
pirouette with the sun 70
pivot
  lower body 95
  pelvic 95
  upper body 94
placement
  head 78
  neck 78
plough 67
positive moves 16
post-viral fatigue syndrome (M.E.) 37, 45
posture 26, 74
power
  ankle 103
  knee 104

lung and heart 109
pregnancy 14
progress chart 134

quarter rolls
    with balance and flop 71
    with kicks 72
    with body curve 73

R.S.I. 37
raw vegetables 51
realignment 71
recovering from a backward bend 115
recovery positions 113
repetitive strain injury (R.S.I.) 37
rises 103
rolling
    board 31
    continuous 73
    quarter rolls with balance and flop 71
    quarter rolls with body curve 73
    quarter rolls with kick 72
roots, back to the 8

S.A.D. (seasonal affective disorder) 45
safe sun-focusing 70
sandwich 125
scarves 28
sciatica 74
sclerosis 65
scoliosis 65
seasonal affective disorder (S.A.D.) 45
sense of balance 19
sense of sight 19
shaking your leg out 102
shirts and ties 28
shoulder
    articulation 97
    bags 28
    joints 90
    pads 28
    placement 77
    stand 68
    throwing off shoulder tension 100
side kicks 93, 108
sitting
    bones 43, 59
    on your own built-in seat 59
    on your heels 8
skeleton 74, 78
slipped disc 74
small jumps 109
'snuggle socks' 32
space
    floor 23
    personal 21
Spanish duet turn 122
specialized movements 11
spinal twist
    horizontal 67
    standing 78

spine 67
    hanging your 101
spinning top 60
spotting your partner's eyes 121, 122
squats 104
stance and balance 74
standing spinal twists 78
standing up 75
stepping up and down 105
strength and endurance 102
stretching 18
    active 91
    passive 16
stretching your hamstrings 83
suits 28
sun-focusing with care 70
surface too high 40
surface too low 40
syndromatic illnesses 21

T'ai chi 13
tampons 28
throwing off upper back and shoulder
        tension 100
Toddlertone 14
toe pulling 81
torso, lengthening 66
trapeze 33
turn
    classic Spanish duet 122
    Dervish 80
turn-in, one-legged 87
turn-out 64, 84
    and turn-in 87
turning
    on the spot 79
    together 120
TV-watching positions 38
twist, horizontal 67

umbrellas 28
upper back and neck loosener 123
upper body pivot 94
upside down co-ordination 111
using body weight rather than force 122
using your feet (in massage) 123

vegetarian 50

watches 28
water retention 55
weight
    body 122
    loss 47, 52
weights, ankle and wrist 32, 109
wobble, wobble, all fall down 60
work station 43
work surfaces 39
wrist and ankle weights 32, 109

yoga 13
Yuri shake 102